CLINICAL CARE CONUNDRUMS

Hospital Medicine: Current Concepts

Scott A. Flanders and Sanjay Saint, *Series Editors*

1. *Inpatient Anticoagulation*
   Margaret C. Fang, Editor
2. *Hospital Images: A Clinical Atlas*
   Paul B. Aronowitz, Editor
3. *Becoming a Consummate Clinician: What Every Student, House Officer and Practitioner Needs to Know*
   Ary L. Goldberger and Zachary D. Goldberger, Editors
4. *Perioperative Medicine: Medical Consultation and Co-Management*
   Amir K. Jaffer and Paul J. Grant, Editors
5. *Clinical Care Conundrums: Challenging Diagnoses in Hospital Medicine*
   James C. Pile, Thomas E. Baudendistel, and Brian J. Harte, Editors

CLINICAL CARE CONUNDRUMS

Challenging Diagnoses in Hospital Medicine

Edited by

JAMES C. PILE, MD
Departments of Hospital Medicine and Infectious Diseases
Cleveland Clinic
Cleveland, Ohio

THOMAS E. BAUDENDISTEL, MD
Department of Medicine
Kaiser Permanente Medical Center
Oakland, California

BRIAN J. HARTE, MD
South Pointe Hospital
Cleveland Clinic Health System
Warrensville Heights, Ohio

Series editors

Scott A. Flanders, M.D., SFHM
Sanjay Saint, M.D., M.PH, FHM

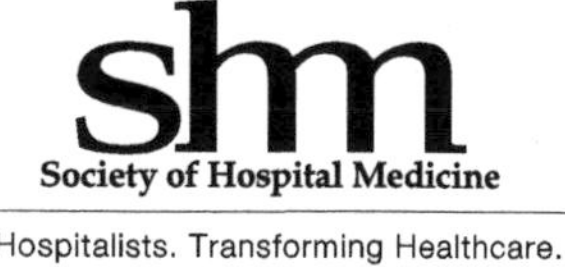

Hospitalists. Transforming Healthcare.
Revolutionizing Patient Care.

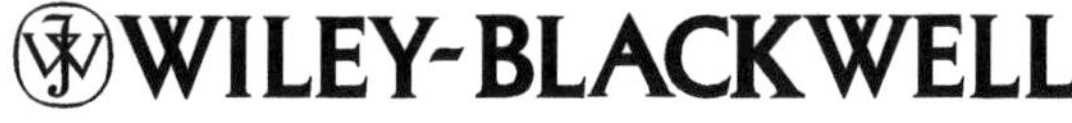

A JOHN WILEY & SONS, INC., PUBLICATION

Wiley Blackwell is an imprint of John Wiley & Sons, formed by the merger of Wiley's global Scientific Technical and Medical business with Blackwell Publishing.

Published by John Wiley & Sons, Inc., Hoboken, New Jersey.
Published simultaneously in Canada.

Library of Congress Cataloging-in-Publication Data:

Pile, James C.
Clinical care conundrums: challenging diagnoses in hospital medicine / James C. Pile, Thomas Baudendistel, Brian Harte.
p.; cm. –(Hospital medicine: current concepts; 7)
Includes bibliographical references.
ISBN 978-0-470-90565-4 (pbk.)
I. Baudendistel, Thomas E. II. Harte, Brian. III. Title. IV. Series: Hospital medicine, current concepts; 7.
[DNLM: 1. Clinical Medicine–methods–Case Reports. 2. Diagnosis, Differential–Case Reports. 3. Evidence-Based Medicine–methods–Case Reports. 4. Hospitalists–Case Reports. WB 293]
616.07′5–dc23

2012030203

Printed in the United States of America

10 9 8 7 6 5 4 3 2 1

CONTENTS

PREFACE

Seven-plus years ago, as planning for the nascent *Journal of Hospital Medicine* was well underway, the journal's inaugural editor-in-chief, Dr. Mark Williams, challenged us to create a feature in which an enigmatic clinical case would be presented in a stepwise manner—in his words, "similar to morning report." With the ultimate diagnosis masked until the end of the case, the Clinical Care Conundrum (CCC) format would allow readers to generate their own hypotheses and differential diagnoses and to compare their thoughts to comments of an expert discussant unfamiliar with the case. Following the unveiling of the diagnosis, a concise discussion would review the key features of the case. We enthusiastically accepted this charge, and over the ensuing years have spent far more hours involved in the endeavor than any of us anticipated at the outset. The bulk of our effort has involved developing relationships with authors and helping them nurture their manuscripts through the review process. Along the way we have found opportunities to coauthor submissions to the feature ourselves. The series has featured manuscripts authored by highly seasoned, senior authors, and we have also had the privilege of working with novice authors and shared their pride in seeing their work in print.

We are proud of the series and consider it a privilege to compile the best of the CCC manuscripts into this book, along with an introductory chapter on clinical reasoning and cognitive error by three experts, Drs. Etchells, Shojania, and Redelmeier. We believe that all the cases in the book will challenge and enhance your diagnostic reasoning skills, and we invite you to use these cases as teaching cases at your institutions.

Building the feature has been a labor of love. We are grateful to a number of individuals, without whose support the series would certainly have been less successful, and in the cases of some, would never have seen the light of publication. First and foremost, we would like to acknowledge Mark Williams, whose vision, good humor, and unfailing support over a number of years were critical to the success of the series. We would also like to thank the *Journal of Hospital Medicine*'s managing editor extraordinaire, Phaedra Cress, whose myriad contributions have been nothing less than remarkable, as well as the journal's current editor, Andy Auerbach, who has continued to support and encourage us in our efforts. Finally, we would be remiss were we not to thank Sanjay Saint and Gurpreet Dhaliwal, both of whom have contributed to the CCC series in a variety of significant ways.

We hope that you enjoy reading the book, and even more importantly, that your patients benefit from you having done so.

Jim Pile, MD
Brian Harte, MD
Tom Baudendistel, MD

January 1, 2013

CONTRIBUTORS

Nima Afshar, MD, Department of Medicine, University of California, San Francisco, California

Makoto Aoki, MD, Sakura Seiki Company, Tokyo, Japan

Wendy Armstrong, MD, Department of Infectious Disease, Emory University School of Medicine, Atlanta, Georgia

Letizia Attala, MD, University of Florence Medical School, Florence, Italy

Jeffrey H. Barsuk, MD, Division of Hospital Medicine, Department of Medicine, Northwestern University Feinberg School of Medicine, Chicago, Illinois

Alessandro Bartoloni, MD, DTM, University of Florence Medical School, Florence, Italy; Tuscan-American Safety Collaborative, Florence, Italy

Thomas E. Baudendistel, MD, FACP, Department of Medicine, Kaiser Permanente Medical Center, Oakland, California

Maytee Boonyapredee, MD, MS, Department of Internal Medicine, Franklin Square Hospital Center, Baltimore, Maryland

Julia Braza, MD, Division of Pathology, Beth Israel Deaconess Medical Center, Harvard Medical School, Boston, Massachusetts

Daniel J. Brotman, MD, FACP, Department of Medicine, Johns Hopkins Hospital, Baltimore, Maryland

Esteban Cheng Ching, MD, Department of Neurology, Cleveland Clinic, Cleveland, Ohio

Sandra Y. Chung, MD, Department of Medicine, University of California, San Francisco, California

Sandro Cinti, MD, Division of Infectious Diseases, Department of Internal Medicine, University of Michigan, Ann Arbor, Michigan

Colin R. Cooke, MD, MSc, Division of Pulmonary and Critical Care Medicine, University of Michigan, Ann Arbor, Michigan

Giampaolo Corti, MD, University of Florence Medical School, Florence, Italy

John Del Valle, MD, Department of Internal Medicine, University of Michigan, Ann Arbor, Michigan

Gurpreet Dhaliwal, MD, Department of Medicine, University of California, San Francisco, California; Medical Service, San Francisco VA Medical Center, San Francisco, California

Louis R. Dibernardo, MD, Department of Pathology, Duke University Medical Center, Duke University, Durham, North Carolina

Julia C. Dombrowski, MD, MPH, Department of Medicine, University of California, San Francisco, California

Edward E. Etchells, MD, MSc, Department of Medicine, Sunnybrook Health Sciences Centre and University of Toronto, Toronto, Ontario, Canada; University of Toronto Centre for Patient Safety, Toronto, Ontario, Canada

Amit Garg, MD, Department of Medicine, Kaiser Permanente Medical Center, Oakland, California

Satish Gopal, MPH, MD, Department of Internal Medicine, Norwalk Hospital, Norwalk, Connecticut

Richard J. Haber, MD, Department of Medicine, University of California, San Francisco, California; Department of Medicine, San Francisco General Hospital, San Francisco, California

Brian J. Harte, MD, FACP, SFHM, South Pointe Hospital, Cleveland Clinic Health System, Warrensville Heights, Ohio

Adrian F. Hernandez, MD, Division of Cardiovascular Medicine, Duke Clinical Research Institute, Duke University Medical Center, Duke University, Durham, North Carolina

Jan V. Hirschmann, MD, Division of General Medicine, Veterans Affairs Puget Sound Health Care System, University of Washington, Seattle, Washington

Harry Hollander, MD, Department of Medicine, University of California, San Francisco, California

Irena L. Ilic, MD, Department of Medicine, Palo Alto Medical Foundation, Palo Alto, California

Aubrey O. Ingraham, MD, Department of Medicine, Kaiser Permanente Medical Center, Oakland, California

S. A. Josephson, MD, Department of Neurology, University of California, San Francisco, California

Saurabh B. Kandpal, MD, Department of Hospital Medicine, Cleveland Clinic, Cleveland, Ohio

Helen Kao, MD, Department of Medicine, University of California, San Francisco, California

Patrick P. Kneeland, MD, Division of Hospital Medicine, Providence Regional Medical Center, Everett, Washington

R. J. Kohlwes, MD, MPH, Department of Medicine, University of California, San Francisco, California

Damon M. Kwan, MD, Division of Cardiology, Kaiser Permanente Medical Center, Los Angeles, California; Department of Medicine, California Pacific Medical Center, San Francisco, California

Benjamin A. Lipsky, MD, Primary and Specialty Medicine Service, Veterans Affairs Puget Sound Health Care System, Department of Medicine, The University of Washington School of Medicine, Seattle, Washington

Jennifer R. Lukela, MD, Department of Internal Medicine, University of Michigan, Ann Arbor, Michigan

Rajesh S. Mangrulkar, MD, Department of Internal Medicine, University of Michigan, Ann Arbor, Michigan

Sara Mekuria, MD, Internal Medicine Residency Program, Cleveland Clinic, Cleveland, Ohio

Satyen Nichani, MD, Division of General Medicine, Department of Internal Medicine, University of Michigan, Ann Arbor, Michigan

Jonathan P. Piccini, MD, Division of Cardiovascular Medicine, Duke Clinical Research Institute, Duke University Medical Center, Duke University, Durham, North Carolina

James C. Pile, MD, FACP, SFHM, Departments of Hospital Medicine and Infectious Diseases, Cleveland Clinic, Cleveland, Ohio

Anuradha Ramaswamy, MD, Department of Hospital Medicine, Cleveland Clinic, Cleveland, Ohio

Ramakrishnan Ranganath, MD, MRCP, Department of Internal Medicine, Franklin Square Hospital Center, Baltimore, Maryland

Gregory J. Raugi, MD, PhD, Primary and Specialty Medicine Service, Veterans Affairs Puget Sound Health Care System, Department of Medicine, The University of Washington School of Medicine, Seattle, Washington

Donald A. Redelmeier, MD, Department of Medicine, Sunnybrook Health Sciences Centre and University of Toronto, Toronto, Ontario, Canada; University of Toronto Centre for Patient Safety, Toronto, Ontario, Canada; Institute for Clinical Evaluative Sciences, Toronto, Ontario, Canada

Natasha Renda, MD, School of Medicine, University of California, San Francisco, California

Joseph G. Rogers, MD, Division of Cardiovascular Medicine, Duke Clinical Research Institute, Duke University Medical Center, Duke University, Durham, North Carolina

Sanjay Saint, MD, MPH, Department of Internal Medicine, University of Michigan, Ann Arbor, Michigan; Ann Arbor VA Health Services Research and Development Field Program, Ann Arbor, Michigan; Patient Safety Enhancement Program, University of Michigan Health System, Ann Arbor, Michigan; Tuscan-American Safety Collaborative, Florence, Italy

Sanjiv J. Shah, MD, Department of Medicine, University of Chicago, Chicago, Illinois; Department of Medicine, University of California, San Francisco, California

John V. L. Sheffield, MD, Division of General Medicine, Harborview Medical Center, University of Washington, Seattle, Washington

Kaveh G. Shojania, MD, Department of Medicine, Sunnybrook Health Sciences Centre and University of Toronto, Toronto, Ontario, Canada; University of Toronto Centre for Patient Safety, Toronto, Ontario, Canada

Gerald W. Smetana, MD, Division of General Medicine and Primary Care, Beth Israel Deaconess Medical Center, Harvard Medical School, Boston, Massachusetts

John Fani Srour, MD, Division of General Medicine and Primary Care, Beth Israel Deaconess Medical Center, Harvard Medical School, Boston, Massachusetts

Jinny Tavee, MD, Department of Neurology, Cleveland Clinic, Cleveland, Ohio

Lawrence M. Tierney, Jr., MD, Department of Medicine, University of California, San Francisco, California

Yasuharu Tokuda, MD, MPH, Department of Medicine, Mito Kyodo General Hospital, University of Tsukuba, Mito City, Japan

Adam Tremblay, MD, Ann Arbor Veterans Affairs Medical Center, University of Michigan, Ann Arbor, Michigan

Robert M. Wachter, MD, Department of Medicine, University of California, San Francisco, California

Jennei Wei, MD, MPH, Department of Medicine, University of California, San Francisco, California

Lisa H. Williams, MD, Primary and Specialty Medicine Service, Veterans Affairs Puget Sound Health Care System, Department of Medicine, The University of Washington School of Medicine, Seattle, Washington

Iris O. Yung, MD, Department of Medicine, California Pacific Medical Center, San Francisco, California

CHAPTER 1

INTRODUCTION TO CLINICAL CARE CONUNDRUMS IN HOSPITAL MEDICINE

ROBERT M. WACHTER

Department of Medicine, University of California, San Francisco, California

One of the challenges of a generalist field—one that cannot define itself by its expertise in managing the derangements of an organ (as with cardiology) or by its skills in performing a procedure (as with surgery)—is to develop a core curriculum and a raison d'être. From the time that Lee Goldman and I coined the term *hospitalist* in 1996,[1] hospitalists began to struggle with this existential question. What was their field about, and what justified its existence?

This struggle abated in 1999–2001, with the publication of two seminal reports on patient safety and healthcare quality by the Institute of Medicine.[2,3] Soon, the hospitalist field had put its collective nickel down: while hospitalists would be excellent doctors in the traditional, Marcus Welbian sense of the word, our unique niche would be as system leaders, helping to build systems to ensure the highest quality, safest care for hospitalized patients.

This focus—which was codified in the publication of the Society of Hospital Medicine's Core Curriculum in 2006[4]—has unquestionably helped the field establish credibility within the House of Medicine and with a variety of important stakeholders, such as legislators, the media, regulators, accreditors, and, most importantly, patients and their advocates. Also, as the overall pressure to improve quality, safety, and value has increased, many hospitals, training programs, and national and international organizations have turned to hospitalists to "see how it is done." This is all for the good—for both patients and for our rapidly growing field.

But, just as we now understand that certain safety fixes can have unanticipated consequences, so too can a narrow focus on systems improvement. I think we have begun to see these consequences play out over the past few years, both as they pertain to our entire system of care and more specifically to the core work of hospitalists.

In 2010, I wrote an article entitled *Why Diagnostic Errors Don't Get Any Respect … and What can be Done About Them*,[5] in which I argued that the focus on systems thinking to address safety targets such as medication errors and falls was terrific, but the crucial matter of diagnostic errors had been strangely omitted from the safety agenda. This "diagnostic errors exceptionalism" began at the beginning, with the IOM report, *To Err is Human*.[2] In that report, the term *medication error* is mentioned 70 times, while the term *diagnostic error* is mentioned fewer than 5 times.

Clinical Care Conundrums: Challenging Diagnoses in Hospital Medicine, First Edition.
Edited by James C. Pile, Thomas E. Baudendistel, and Brian J. Harte.

However, diagnostic errors make up nearly one in five preventable adverse events in the famous Harvard Medical Practice Study[6] and they are far more common than medication errors in studies of closed malpractice claims.[7]

It is easy to see why diagnostic errors have been overlooked in the safety field: they are hard to measure and fix. But by ignoring them, we risk a self-fulfilling prophesy, one in which we get better in developing process changes, information technology, and checklists that address system errors, while neglecting interventions and research that could ultimately improve diagnostic accuracy.

Luckily, diagnostic errors have recently started to receive the attention they deserve, from academic experts, accrediting boards, and researchers.[8–10] Also, some promising solutions are beginning to emerge, both in the form of new ways of thinking (such as metacognition and cognitive de-biasing)[11] and in new models of computerized decision support.[12] But even with these methods, I believe that the time-honored tradition of having clinicians learn from tough cases remains central to our efforts to improve diagnostic reasoning.

This brings me to the more specific issue for hospitalists. While the American hospitalist model has taken on unique aspects, the US hospitalist in some regards resembles the Canadian or British internist—a hospital-based highly trained physician who specializes in managing the really knotty cases that have stumped everyone else. In America, we know what such a doctor looks like: Dr. Gregory House (hopefully without the arrogance, inappropriateness, and substance abuse). Andrew Holtz, in his 2006 book, "The Medical Science of House," recognized this.[13] "Although Dr. House is called a 'diagnostician,' he is really a hospitalist," wrote Holtz. While we have focused on the hospitalist as systems improver, the need for a "go-to" diagnostician remains, and hospitalists have assumed this role in many of their institutions, not just on television.

Perhaps in the distant future, a computer—maybe a version of IBM's Jeopardy-beating computer Watson—will obviate the need for a really smart physician, willing and able to gather all the relevant facts and armed with the experience and training required to convert these facts into a differential diagnosis, a diagnostic plan, and ultimately the right diagnosis. But today, we depend on physicians to serve in this role. To excel as a diagnostician, we know that clinicians need to constantly mine both their own cases as well as the cases of others for lessons. It would be best if these learning cases were carefully selected for their lessons, and if one could follow the thinking of a master clinician as he or she worked through their cognitive twists and turns.

All of which is to say that the lessons contained in this book are crucial for hospitalists if we are going to fulfill our dual missions of being system improvers and superb diagnosticians. I suspect you will read it, then return to it over and over through the years for wisdom and inspiration.

REFERENCES

1. Wachter RM, Goldman L. The emerging role of "hospitalists" in the American health care system. *New Engl J Med*. 1996;335:514–517.
2. Kohn L, Corrigan J, Donaldson M, eds. *To Err is Human: Building a Safer Health System*. Washington, DC: Committee on Quality of Health Care in America, Institute of Medicine. National Academy Press; 2000.
3. Committee on Quality of Health Care in America, IOM. *Crossing the quality chasm: a new health system for the 21st century*. Washington, DC: National Academy Press; 2001.
4. McKean SC, Budnitz TL, Dressler DD, Amin AN, Pistoria MJ. How to use the core competencies in hospital medicine: a framework for curriculum development. *J Hosp Med*. 2006;1:57–67.

5. Wachter RM. Why diagnostic errors don't get any respect... and what can be done about them. *Health Aff*. 2010;29:1605–1610.
6. Leape LL, Brennan TA, Laird N, et al. The nature of adverse events in hospitalized patients. Results of the Harvard Medical Practice Study II. *N Engl J Med*. 1991;324:377–384.
7. Bishop TF, Ryan AK, Casalino LP. Paid malpractice claims for adverse events in inpatient and outpatient settings. *JAMA*. 2011;305:2427–2431.
8. Newman-Toker DE, Pronovost PJ. Diagnostic errors–the next frontier for patient safety. *JAMA*. 2009;301:1060–1062.
9. Redelmeier DA. Improving patient care. The cognitive psychology of missed diagnoses. *Ann Intern Med*. 2005;142:115–120.
10. Groopman J. *How doctors think*. Boston, MA: Houghton Mifflin; 2007.
11. Croskerry P. The importance of cognitive errors in diagnosis and strategies to minimize them. *Acad Med*. 2003;78:775–780.
12. Ramnarayan P, Cronje N, Brown R, et al. Validation of a diagnostic reminder system in emergency medicine: a multi-centre study. *Emerg Med J*. 2007;24:619–624.
13. Holtz A. *The medical science of House, M.D*. New York: Berkley Trade; 2006.

CHAPTER 2

IMPROVING DIAGNOSTIC SAFETY IN HOSPITAL MEDICINE: CAN CLINICAL CARE CONUNDRUMS HELP?

EDWARD E. ETCHELLS and KAVEH G. SHOJANIA

Department of Medicine, Sunnybrook Health Sciences Centre and University of Toronto, Toronto, Ontario, Canada; University of Toronto Centre for Patient Safety, Toronto, Ontario, Canada

DONALD A. REDELMEIER

Department of Medicine, Sunnybrook Health Sciences Centre and University of Toronto, Toronto, Ontario, Canada; University of Toronto Centre for Patient Safety, Toronto, Ontario, Canada; Institute for Clinical Evaluative Sciences, Toronto, Ontario, Canada

INTRODUCTION

One of us (EE) recently read a "Clinical Care Conundrum" in the *Journal of Hospital Medicine* that described a 45-year-old female patient with recurrent unexplained delirium.[1] The final diagnosis was Hashimoto's encephalopathy. EE was fascinated. He had never heard of this diagnosis being mentioned in any consultation, conversation, lecture, morning report, rounds, article, chapter, monograph, or text. For the next few months, every time EE heard about a delirious patient, the diagnosis of Hashimoto's encephalopathy popped into his mind. He made a special point of mentioning the diagnosis at morning report and during case discussions, hoping to look intelligent. His coauthors (KGS and DAR) thought that EE was becoming increasingly tangential and wondered if his reading the clinical conundrum had been helpful or harmful.

In this chapter, we

1. describe the frequency and consequences of diagnostic delay and diagnosis-related harm;
2. analyze causes of diagnostic delay and diagnosis-related harm;
3. review core concepts in diagnostic reasoning and common cognitive errors;
4. outline steps that might improve diagnostic safety in hospital medicine.

Clinical Care Conundrums: Challenging Diagnoses in Hospital Medicine, First Edition.
Edited by James C. Pile, Thomas E. Baudendistel, and Brian J. Harte.

DIAGNOSTIC DELAY AND DIAGNOSIS-RELATED HARM

Diagnosis is the process of knowing (Greek, *gnosis*) through separating (*dia* = apart) the clinical findings in a patient. Diagnosis can be conceptualized as a process of managing and reducing uncertainty, while minimizing the potential for patient harm.[2] The hospitalist may be less concerned about the correct final diagnosis, provided all dangerous causes of the patient's presenting syndrome are rapidly considered and excluded. For a patient with nausea and vomiting, the hospitalist will want to rapidly evaluate common serious possibilities, such as acute myocardial infarction (MI). The hospitalist may be willing to accept uncertainty about less harmful causes of nausea and vomiting, such as gastritis. A final precise diagnosis may not be reached during hospitalization.[3] Even after an exhaustive diagnostic evaluation, many common clinical syndromes, such as syncope and delirium in the elderly, often defy a precise diagnosis.[4,5]

Diagnostic delay (or diagnostic error) can be defined as a diagnosis that was delayed despite the availability of sufficient information to make the diagnosis, as judged from the eventual appreciation of more definitive information.[6] We favor the term *diagnostic delay* rather than diagnostic error for two reasons. First, most diagnoses are ultimately made, but could have been made sooner. Second, some diagnoses are initially obscure despite vigorous diagnostic efforts. In such cases, it may not be possible to identify a diagnostic delay or error, even though the initial diagnostic impressions ultimately proved wrong.

There are relatively few prospective studies of diagnostic delay in hospitalist practice. One prospective study found that junior residents working in a medical intensive care unit or coronary unit experienced about 19 diagnostic errors with substantial potential to cause harm per 1000 patient days, during an 80-hour workweek. Assuming each resident cares for 10 patients per day, this translates into 1 serious diagnostic error per resident per week.[7]

Diagnosis-related harm can be defined as preventable harm that results from the delay or failure to treat a condition actually present or from treatment provided for a condition not actually present.[8] Several large retrospective chart review studies found diagnosis-related harm in 0.3%–2.2% of all hospital admissions, representing about 4%–15% of all adverse events. About 20%–45% of diagnosis-related harms are associated with permanent disability or death. Diagnosis-related harms are more likely to be judged preventable (80%) compared to other types of adverse events (25%–50%).[9–13] Approximately 75,000 US hospital admissions per year are due to diagnosis-related harm.[14] Diagnosis-related harm is an important cause of medicolegal claims, accounting for about 60% of emergency department and ambulatory care claims.[15,16]

Autopsy is an important method for detecting diagnosis-related harm. There are unsuspected important diagnoses detected in 8%–24% of autopsies; in 3%–6% of autopsies, the unsuspected diagnosis contributed to death.[17]

Most delayed diagnoses involve common conditions. The top five final diagnoses in a large study of diagnostic delay in internal medicine were pulmonary embolism, drug reaction, lung cancer, colorectal cancer, and acute coronary syndrome.[18] The most common diagnostic delay in an emergency department setting was a missed fracture.[19] These studies highlight the importance of appreciating base-rate probabilities when forming diagnostic hypotheses and provide empirical support for the diagnostic aphorism "when you hear hoof beats, think horses not zebras."

Clinicians rely heavily on diagnostic test information, yet diagnostic tests are also susceptible to error. About 18% of critical laboratory results are judged nonrepresentative of the patient's clinical condition after a chart review, likely reflecting errors related to specimen collection and handling.[20] CT scans have 1.7% misinterpretation rate.[21] Pathologic discrepancies occur in 11%–19% of cancer biopsy specimens.[22,23] These data should remind clinicians to question laboratory and pathologic results that are discordant with the rest of the patient's clinical picture.

Diagnostic delays stem from cognitive factors, system factors, and their interaction. A recent retrospective study evaluated the causes of 100 diagnostic delays assembled from autopsy series, quality assurance reviews, and voluntary physician reports.[6] Both cognitive and system factors contributed to 46% of cases, while 28% involved only cognitive factors and 19%, only system factors. A minority (7%) of cases were classified as "no fault" due to unusual disease presentations. A similar pattern of cognitive and system contributors was identified when the Diagnosis Error Evaluation and Research (DEER) classification system was applied to over 500 diagnostic errors.[18]

DIAGNOSTIC REASONING AND COGNITIVE ERRORS

Cognition contributes to about 75% of diagnosis-related harms. According to the dual processing theory of diagnostic reasoning, there are two distinct problem-solving modes: intuitive and analytic.[24] The clinician facing a diagnostic problem intuitively searches for a recognizable pattern, such as when a clinician hears a description of crushing retrosternal chest pain and the diagnosis of MI comes to mind. If no pattern is recognized, then analytic thinking is activated, typically as hypothesis generation. After generating three to seven hypotheses, the analytic process will usually stop until new information is available.[25] For the patient with chest pain, hypotheses might include pneumonia, pericarditis, and aortic dissection. In some cases, the clinician may not be able to generate even a single hypothesis for an unusual problem. In such situations, exhaustive data gathering and consultation may be required. This exhaustive approach might be used by an experienced clinician facing an unusual problem, such as a patient who is complaining of an unusual crunching sound during eye movement and vertigo induced by loud noises.

Both intuitive and analytic thinking serve clinicians and patients well. Although the analytic approach is congruent with the iconic image of an Oslerian clinical detective, there is no evidence that hypothesis generation is inherently more accurate than intuitive pattern recognition, for experts or novices.[26] EKG interpretation by complete novices was more accurate if they were encouraged to both use their instincts and apply analytic rules, compared to novices who were primed to use only one problem-solving method.[27]

The analytic and intuitive thinking modes can be simultaneously active, providing a cross-checking function. Such cross-checking might be suppressed by many system factors, such as fatigue or hunger. The rate of serious diagnostic delay by residents was reduced from 19 to 3 serious diagnostic errors per 1000 patient days with restriction of work hours from 85 to 64 hours per week.[7] Similarly, study participants who ingested glucose-based lemonade activated more analytic thinking on functional MRI than a control group who consumed lemonade sweetened with sugar substitute.[28]

Calibration is the degree to which diagnostic confidence and diagnostic accuracy agree. Clinician's decisions were poorly calibrated in a study of difficult internal medicine paper cases. Overall, clinicians listed the correct diagnosis in their differentials for 40% of the cases, reflecting the difficulty of the cases.[29] Clinicians were confident that they had the correct diagnosis 30% of the time, reflecting an appropriate degree of diagnostic humility. Of concern, when clinicians were confident that they were correct, they were correct only 68% of the time. If clinicians were not confident, they were still correct 29% of the time. This poor calibration between "confidence" and "correctness" was seen in both residents and staff physicians.

There are several characteristics of expert diagnostic thinking.[26,30] First, experts use both intuitive thinking and analytic thinking. Clinicians, educators, and students must all acknowledge and embrace intuitive problem solving, rather than avoid or reject it. The way to develop intuitive problem solving is to see many patients and follow-up until the final diagnosis is established.[31] Second, experts intuitively recognize more patterns and do so more efficiently. In one study, six expert dermatologists reviewing 100 skin lesion photographs were 86% accurate and gave correct answers within 8 seconds, whereas medical students were only 21% accurate and gave their (few) correct answers within 12 seconds.[32] Third, intuitive pattern recognition expertise is content specific. One hospitalist may have considerable expertise for distinguishing patterns of third nerve palsies, yet that same hospitalist might be unable to correctly recognize a vesiculobullous skin eruption. Fourth, experts are more skilled at many aspects of analytical thinking. Experts correctly interpret limited clinical data more often, and more efficiently, than nonexperts.[33]

Once a diagnostic impression has formed, the clinician's challenge is to keep an open mind as the clinical situation unfolds. The diagnostic process must be revisited, revised, or reopened as new information appears. Reopening can be due to either rational Bayesian principles, such as a series of nondiagnostic test results, or clinical red flags, such as deterioration in the patient's status. Unfortunately, there are entrenched cognitive processes that can potentially keep the clinician's mind closed.[34]

Heuristics and Metacognition

There are well-defined cognitive processes, or heuristics, that are routinely used for problem solving. Hospitalists should have a working knowledge of common cognitive heuristics for at least three reasons. First, knowledge of heuristics may allow one to correct one's own errors in thought. Such cognitive self-awareness is termed *metacognition*. Second, even if one cannot correct one's own errors in thinking, knowledge of heuristics may allow identification of such errors in a colleague's thinking. Finally, knowledge of heuristics helps to normalize, rather than vilify, cognitive diagnostic error, so that such errors can be discussed in a nonpunitive learning environment.

The label of cognitive bias is often applied when a heuristic has negative consequences. The indiscriminate use of the label cognitive bias is unjustified because many heuristics facilitate efficient and accurate problem solving.[36] We will focus on two major cognitive heuristics (Table 2.1). There are recent reviews with full descriptions of many other heuristics and biases.[37,38]

The first cognitive heuristic is the tendency to stop diagnostic thinking once an initial impression has been formed, without further consideration of alternative possibilities. This diagnostic efficiency is not necessarily a bad thing. Experienced clinicians stop data gathering and draw conclusions well before all possible data are collected, yet retain accuracy. A good predictor of diagnostic success is the early appearance of the correct diagnosis on the list of hypotheses.[36] Additional information is not necessarily helpful. In one study, expert clinicians had better diagnostic accuracy when viewing photographs with no other information, compared to viewing photographs and receiving additional verbal clinical information.[39]

TABLE 2.1 Heuristics, Biases, and Metacognitive Remedies

Heuristic	What We Call It When It Fails Us ("Cognitive Bias")	Proposed Metacognitive Questions to Help Prevent Bias	Important Educational Topics to Reduce Error[35]
Only collect as much information as necessary to solve a problem	Premature closure	What else could it be?	Bayesian knowledge Highly specific features (for quick rule-ins) Highly sensitive features (for quick rule-outs) Red flag alerts for clinical syndromes Checklists of core information for solving common clinical problems
	Confirmation bias	How would I interpret this information if it was available when I first saw the patient? What clinical data would prove me wrong?	Bayesian knowledge Highly specific features (for quick rule-ins) Highly sensitive features (for quick rule-outs)
	Framing bias	What if I reframed this case as not yet diagnosed?	Confirm with the patient why they came to hospital and what is bothering them Include level of certainty in diagnostic summaries and handovers Avoid or ignore emotion-laden terms
Pattern recognition is influenced by ease of recall of prior similar cases	Availability bias	Am I merely remembering my most recent similar case?	Base-rate knowledge

Unfortunately, if the correct diagnosis is not on the initial list, diagnostic delay is more likely to occur. In such cases, this heuristic then becomes a "bias," most commonly referred to as *premature closure*. Premature closure accounts for almost half of the cognitive biases identified in studies of diagnostic error, possibly because there are several related cognitive processes that promote premature closure. First, clinicians tend to seek out information that supports their initial diagnostic impressions (confirmation bias). Medical students overwhelmingly sought nondiagnostic data that fit their initial impressions; only 17% of students correctly sought further information that could distinguish the two major diagnostic possibilities.[40] Second, clinicians tend to overvalue irrelevant information if it has been deliberately sought after.[41] Third, information that supports initial impressions is overvalued, while information that conflicts with initial impressions is downplayed or ignored (anchoring bias). Anchoring may explain why patients persist in the belief that their arthritis symptoms correlate with weather, even when no such correlation exists.[42] Finally, clinicians tend to stick to initial impressions as the number of new possibilities increases (complexity bias). Physicians were more likely to stick with their current plan when confronted with two additional therapeutic options as opposed to being confronted with only one additional therapeutic option.[43]

Premature closure can be further exacerbated by framing effects. These "framing" effects can include overreliance on another clinician's hypothesis, failure to communicate uncertainty, and emotional reactions to diagnostically irrelevant variables. If an emergency physician refers "a 65-year-old patient with pneumonia," a very small cognitive frame has been placed around the patient's problem. If the same patient is referred as "a 65-year-old patient with a 1-day history of dyspnea, fever, and chest pain," there is a broader diagnostic frame that allows for broader diagnostic thinking ("Could this be pulmonary embolism or pericarditis?").

The magnitude of framing effects can be large. In one study, patients, graduate students, and doctors ($n = 1153$) considered a hypothetical scenario where they faced a choice between surgery and radiation treatment for lung cancer. Participants randomly received the surgical treatment in a mortality frame (10% chance of death) and a survival frame (90% chance of survival). Although both options are identical, the subtle change in wording had a profound effect on decision making. With the mortality frame, only 58% chose surgery, whereas with the survival frame 75% chose surgery.[44] In another study, physicians were more likely to list coronary heart disease as their initial impression for a chest pain scenario, if the scenario was framed by the statement that another doctor thought that the patient might have coronary heart disease.[45] Subtle wording can also have important but unintended framing effects. Emotional but diagnostically irrelevant terms, such as *bounce back*, should be avoided or discounted during the diagnostic process.

The second large cognitive heuristic is that intuitive thinking is dominated by ease of recall of past similar cases. This "availability heuristic" is useful for busy clinicians seeing common presentations of common conditions. Unfortunately, the availability heuristic can create problems when a hospitalist encounters an uncommon cause of a common syndrome. If your last patient with acute nontraumatic chest pain had an aortic dissection, you will tend to think of aortic dissection in the next few patients with chest pain, even though MI is much more common. A 75-year-old man with sudden-onset dyspnea and hemoptysis, EKG findings of acute right heart strain, and CXR findings of segmental oligemia, and a peripheral wedge-shaped consolidation (Hampton's hump) almost certainly has a pulmonary embolism, but this pattern of signs and symptoms is unusual.[46] The ease of recall of the dramatic but unusual presentation may lead the clinician away from the diagnosis of pulmonary embolism in the next patient with a typical, but less dramatic, presentation.

Irrelevant but easily recalled clinical features can unduly influence diagnostic thinking. In an intriguing study, medical residents were taught the EKG features of acute anterior MI. In one group, the teaching case was a 51-year-old male; in the second group, the teaching case was identical except it was a 51-year-old male banker. All participants were then asked to interpret the EKG of a 51-year-old banker with chest pain and a left bundle branch block that did not meet criteria for diagnosing MI. Residents in the first ("no banker") group correctly diagnosed NO MI 46% of the time, whereas residents in the second ("banker") group correctly diagnosed NO MI only 23% of the time. The ease of recall of the patient's profession, an irrelevant clinical feature, led many residents to incorrectly diagnose acute MI.[47]

IMPROVING DIAGNOSTIC SAFETY AND ACCURACY

Diagnostic safety should improve within a culture that accepts, learns from, and trains clinicians to reduce diagnostic error, and by implementation of systematic methods to reduce and trap diagnostic error.

There are insufficient studies to make strong evidence-based recommendations for individual and system improvements for diagnostic safety. Diagnostic safety studies often involve hypothetical paper cases rather than real patients on hospital wards. Improvement strategies derived solely from such studies may not be applicable to the hospital medicine setting. We propose 13 strategies, while acknowledging that further study is needed (Tables 2.2 and 2.3).

Read Clinical Care Conundrums Wisely

Clinical problem-solving manuscripts such as Clinical Care Conundrums might improve diagnostic safety by promoting a learning culture where difficult, or erroneous, diagnostic processes are shared and analyzed. Clinical Care Conundrums can also be a useful method for learning and applying diagnostic safety principles (Table 2.3). Readers should avoid excessive focus on the final diagnosis, since these manuscripts tend to focus on rarer conditions.

Learn Diagnostic Red Flags

A diagnostic red flag signals the clinician to reopen the diagnostic process, thus jarring the brain out of potentially premature closure. Diagnostic red flags can be nonspecific, such as deterioration in the patient's status, or specific to a clinical syndrome or differential diagnosis. For example, if your colleague does not mention the blood pressure in both arms for the patient with acute nontraumatic chest pain, a specific red flag should go up because your colleague may not have considered aortic dissection. Unexplained symptoms or findings also represent diagnostic red flags. For instance, a patient with chest pain is admitted to rule out an acute coronary syndrome. Cardiac biomarkers are negative, but the patient's white blood count is slightly elevated. Focusing on this unexplained abnormality can prompt the clinician to ask the patient more carefully about the

TABLE 2.2 Improving Diagnostic Safety and Accuracy

1.	Read clinical conundrums wisely
2.	Learn diagnostic red flags
3.	Involve your patients
4.	Share your thinking
5.	Share your uncertainty
6.	Foster a culture of diagnostic safety
7.	Enhance diagnostic feedback
8.	Promote teamwork
9.	Create and test diagnostic checklists
10.	Explore automated diagnostic systems
11.	Make diagnostic reports user friendly
12.	Implement reliable follow-up systems
13.	Conduct prospective diagnostic safety research "On The Wards"

TABLE 2.3 Using Clinical Care Conundrums to Learn and Apply Diagnostic Safety Principles

Diagnostic Safety Principle	Learning Method
Know base-rate probabilities to avoid availability bias	After the opening paragraph, list three to seven common causes of the patient's presenting problem Compare your list with that of the expert clinician to see where and why they diverge Describe baseline probabilities for these common conditions
Keep an open mind to avoid premature closure	List three to seven less common causes of the patient's presenting problem As subsequent information is presented, add new diagnoses and remove ones you no longer feel are likely. See how your reordering matches with that of the discussant
Apply Bayesian principles	Decide whether new information warrants a change in diagnostic thinking based on Bayesian principles Did you (or the discussant) give appropriate weight to diagnostic information? If not, why? Learning the sensitivity and specificity of this new diagnostic information can enhance diagnostic safety and accuracy
Avoid confirmation bias and framing effects	As new information appears, ask: "What else could this be?" "What wouldn't I want to miss at this point?"
Calibrate your diagnostic thinking	Describe how lessons from this clinical conundrum will be applied to your next patient with a similar clinical presentation If the final diagnosis from this clinical conundrum pops into mind, consider whether availability bias is unduly influencing your thought process

quality of his or her pain and to reinspect the EKGs looking for changes in the ST or PR segments suggestive of pericarditis.

Involve Your Patients

The patient is the central figure in all diagnostic activity, yet the patient's voice can be hidden behind laboratory data, radiology reports, and paperwork. Patients have a much shorter roster of concerns than doctors and may be paying more attention to their specific case. Hospitalists should encourage and welcome questions about the diagnostic thinking, including diagnostic uncertainty, from their patients. The National Patient Safety Foundation has a diagnostic safety checklist for patients, including asking the doctor "What else could this be?"[48] Well-informed patients might reduce the risk of diagnostic delay when the clinical condition remains uncertain. If a patient with subacute back pain is told to watch for the red flags of spinal cord compression, subtle changes in urinary function or gait might be identified and evaluated more quickly.

Share Your Thinking

Cognitive self-awareness (metacognition) may help strike the balance between valuable heuristics and harmful biases. Several metacognitive remedies have been proposed, although the effectiveness of these remedies has not been fully evaluated. To combat premature closure, clinicians can ask themselves "What else could it be?" The strongest remedies for availability and confirmation bias are knowledge of the base rate (prevalence) of common clinical diagnoses and of the diagnostic accuracy of clinical examination data.[49]

It can be hard to monitor one's own thought processes while one is in the midst of thinking. However, cognitive self-awareness can also be activated when discussing a patient with a colleague. An effective discussion can highlight the clinician's thought processes, including positive findings with high specificity ("rule-ins"), as well as the negative findings with high sensitivity ("rule-outs").[50] Consider the following handover from an emergency room physician to your hospitalist service: "I am admitting a 65 year old with a provisional diagnosis of community acquired pneumonia. The presenting complaints were fever, cough, and chest pain. The chest X-ray showed an alveolar infiltrate in the left lower lobe." This well-framed handover allows the receiving hospitalist to understand the initial thought process, generate additional hypotheses, and ask questions.

Share Your Uncertainty

Sharing diagnostic uncertainty allows colleagues to endorse or challenge the diagnostic process. Suppose one hospitalist describes a new admission to a colleague as follows: "I have some uncertainty about the diagnosis for the patient with a low jugular venous pulse, a negative hepatojugular reflex, minimal leg edema, bibasilar crackles, and pulmonary edema on the chest film; my provisional diagnosis is decompensated heart failure, but it doesn't all fit." A colleague might challenge the data integration and synthesis, so that other possibilities, such as lymphangitic carcinomatosis, are considered. In cases with significant uncertainty, it may be better to avoid exact diagnostic labels. If a patient has unexplained chest pain, an admitting diagnosis of unexplained chest pain may be preferable to an admitting diagnosis of possible costochondritis. The diagnosis of unexplained chest pain better frames the diagnostic uncertainty. Furthermore, the word "possible" can easily be omitted during subsequent handovers, leaving the patient with an incorrect diagnostic label of costochondritis.

Foster a Culture of Diagnostic Safety

A culture of diagnostic safety accepts that diagnostic delay is not only inevitable but also a valuable learning opportunity. A hospitalist service with a culture of safety will have regular "safety rounds," during which diagnostic delays are discussed in a supportive learning environment. This service will accept that many diagnostic delays might appear to be individual problems, yet the solutions will always go beyond the individual. This service will ensure that its members (including residents and students for teaching services) know when diagnostic delay is identified and will be evaluated based on their response to the delay rather than the delay itself. An excellent response will include (i) taking necessary steps to reduce the potential for harm to the patient, (ii) presenting the case for discussion and analysis, (iii) proposing individual and system methods that could reduce the potential for future delays, and (iv) participating in disclosure to the patient and family, when appropriate. This safe hospitalist service will identify and mitigate system factors that can increase the likelihood of diagnostic delay, such as excessive workload, long work hours, or poorly constructed information systems.

Enhance Diagnostic Feedback

Feedback is central to development of expertise. Chess players receive immediate and salient feedback each time they lose a piece or suffer a checkmate. By contrast, diagnostic feedback for hospitalists is inconsistent and ambiguous. Suppose a discharged patient does not come back to the emergency department during the next week. Should this patient be considered a diagnostic success or a diagnostic failure? This lack of feedback is a serious threat to the development of diagnostic expertise.

Without feedback, hospitalists can fall into a cycle of false confirmation, misplaced confidence, and poor diagnostic calibration. Better feedback may enhance expertise, help achieve better calibration of diagnostic thinking, improve the educational experience, and intercept diagnostic delays before harm occurs.[3] Salient diagnostic feedback will focus on the relevant aspects of the diagnostic process for common serious conditions.[2,51] Suppose a patient with recurrent pneumonia turns out to have drug-induced pneumonitis. Good feedback will highlight the importance of a history of amiodarone therapy rather than focusing on failure to record the same patient's irrelevant plantar responses.

There may be systematic ways to enhance diagnostic feedback on a hospitalist service. Patients who have experienced a diagnostic delay could be identified by triggers, such as transfers to a higher level of care, or unplanned readmissions. Increasing autopsy rates could improve diagnostic feedback.[17] Electronic clinical documentation can facilitate sharing of diagnostic uncertainty and feedback across the many transitions in care.[52]

Promote Teamwork

Teamwork can probably detect and correct diagnostic errors, although this is an underexplored area in diagnostic safety. Residents faced with diagnostic or therapeutic uncertainty will consult with colleagues or staff for help, while failure to seek such help can lead to delay and harm.[53] Teamwork extends to consultant services, the clinical laboratory, the radiology department, and other areas where diagnostic activity occurs. When the diagnosis is unclear, face-to-face discussions can be rewarding.

Create and Test Diagnostic Checklists

Checklists improve the safety of clinical procedures, such as central line insertions.[54] Evidence-based diagnostic checklists could promote diagnostic safety, particularly when integrated into an electronic clinical record. A simple checklist for diagnosis of altered mental status could help a hospitalist remember to check the capillary blood glucose level. When admitting a patient with unexplained dysphagia, a sophisticated diagnostic checklist could remind the clinician to assess for an exaggerated jaw jerk (for pseudobulbar palsy) and neck extensor weakness (for myasthenia gravis). Exhaustive checklists that are not targeted to the current problem will probably be less effective. A jaw jerk item on an acute chest pain checklist will justifiably be ignored.

Explore Automated Diagnostic Systems

Several computer-assisted diagnostic systems have been developed over the past 30 years. Initial efforts were disappointing,[55,56] but more recent systems have provided more encouraging results. One system correctly listed the diagnosis for 96% ($N = 50$) of *New England Journal of Medicine* "Case Records of the Massachusetts General Hospital" when selected key words were entered by an internist, although the internist using the system was aware of the final correct diagnosis. When the entire Case Record text was entered via a simple cut and paste, the correct diagnosis appeared in a list of 30 suggested diagnoses 76% of the time, although it listed within the top 10 results for only 38% of cases with data entry requiring less than a minute.[57] The incremental value of computerized diagnostic systems over usual clinical decision making remains unknown.

Make Diagnostic Reports User Friendly

Normal and alarming diagnostic reports can appear surprisingly similar, and the concerning diagnostic data can be lost in a sea of irrelevant data. A critically reduced aortic valve area can be buried among uninterpretable diastolic function parameters on an echocardiogram report. Synoptic reporting that both standardizes the display of results and ensures the visibility and review of concerning features can help clinicians to register and interpret important results.[58]

Implement Reliable Communication Systems

Even if laboratory and radiology results are correct and easily readable, the results must reach clinicians. Critical laboratory values do not reach the ordering provider about 2% of the time.[59] Diagnostic test results are not followed up for 20%–60% of patients after discharge.[60] A safe and reliable postdischarge follow-up system that brings new information to the attention of the responsible provider(s) can probably mitigate these errors. An automated system of alerting outpatient physicians to critical radiology results was associated with a very low (0.2%) rate of critical radiology results that were lost to follow-up. The ideal design of these systems remains to be established. In the automated radiology follow-up system, 35% of the alerts were never acknowledged by the receiving clinicians.[61] In another study, 48% of clinicians never used a computerized system designed to bring postdischarge results to the attention of the discharging physician.[62]

Conduct Prospective Diagnostic Safety Research on Hospitalist Services

There are relatively few studies of the diagnostic process as it unfolds in the inpatient practice.[2,51] Hospitalists should open their wards and their thought processes for study. There is a lack of prospective studies that examine cognitive and systemic factors related to diagnostic errors. We cannot understand the problem, or design ideal solutions, based solely on artificial paper-based cases or retrospective recall of memorable diagnostic misadventures. We hope that in the next edition of this book, the section on Reduction of Diagnostic Error might be larger than the section on Causes of Diagnostic Error.

CONCLUSION

EE revised his lessons from the clinical conundrum of the 45-year-old with recurrent unexplained delirium. His first lesson was that recurrent delirium in a patient younger than 65 years is a diagnostic red flag that warrants analytic thinking. Neurologic consultation should be sought if a diagnosis is not identified, even if the patient improves. The second lesson he learnt was that when Hashimoto's encephalopathy pops into mind, be aware of the availability heuristic. Hashimoto's encephalopathy is rare, so there should be other clinical features, such as a family history of autoimmune endocrinopathy or an enlarged thyroid gland, to consider before pursuing the diagnosis.

After about 5 months, EE saw a young patient with vitiligo, pernicious anemia, and an unexplained delirium. The antimicrosomal antibodies were significantly elevated. A diagnosis of Hashimoto's encephalopathy was made, a diagnosis that would not have been possible without the help of the clinical conundrum.

REFERENCES

1. Mekuria S, Ching EC, Josephson SA, Tavee J, Harte BJ. The third time's the charm. *J Hosp Med*. 2009;4:515–520.
2. Crandall B, Wears RL. Expanding perspectives on misdiagnosis. *Am J Med*. 2008;121(5A):S30–S33.
3. Schiff GD. Minimizing diagnostic error: the importance of follow-up and feedback. *Am J Med*. 2008;121(5A):S38–S42.
4. Strickberger SA, Benson DW, Biaggioni I, et al. AHA/ACCF scientific statement on the evaluation of syncope. *Circulation*. 2006;113:316–327.
5. Inouye SK. Delirium in older persons. *N Engl J Med*. 2006;354:1157–1165.
6. Graber ML, Franklin N, Gordon R. Diagnostic error in internal medicine. *Arch Intern Med*. 2005;165:1493–1499.
7. Landrigan CP, Rothschild JM, Cronin JW, et al. Effect of reducing interns' work hours on serious medical errors in intensive care units. *N Engl J Med*. 2004;351:1838–1848.
8. Newman-Toker DE, Pronovost PJ. Diagnostic errors—the next frontier for patient safety. *JAMA*. 2009;301:1060–1062.
9. Baker GR, Norton PG, Flintoft V, et al. The Canadian adverse events study: the incidence of adverse events among hospital patients in Canada. *CMAJ*. 2004;170:1678–1686.
10. Wilson RM, Runciman WB, Gibberd RW, Harrison BT, Newby L, Hamilton JD. The quality in Australian health care study. *Med J Aust*. 1995;163:458–476.
11. Leape LL, Brennan TA, Laird N, et al. The nature of adverse events in hospitalized patients. Results of the Harvard Medical Practice Study II. *N Engl J Med*. 1991;324:377–384.
12. Thomas EJ, Studdert DM, Burstin HR, et al. Incidence and types of adverse events and negligent care in Utah and Colorado. *Med Care*. 2000;38:261–271.
13. Zwaan L, de Bruijne M, Wagner C, et al. Patient record review of the incidence, consequences, and causes of diagnostic adverse events. *Arch Intern Med*. 2010;170:1015–1021.
14. Woods DM, Thomas EJ, Holl JL, Weiss KB, Brennan TA. Ambulatory care adverse events and preventable adverse events leading to a hospital admission. *Qual Saf Health Care*. 2007;16:127–131.
15. Kachalia A, Gandhi TK, Puopolo AL, et al. Missed and delayed diagnoses in the emergency department: a study of closed malpractice claims from 4 liability insurers. *Ann Emerg Med*. 2007;49:196–205.
16. Katz HP, Kaltsounis D, Halloran L, Mondor M. Patient safety and telephone medicine: some lessons from closed claim case review. *J Gen Intern Med*. 2008;23:517–522.
17. Shojania KG, Burton EC, McDonald KM, Goldman L. Changes in rates of autopsy-detected diagnostic errors over time: a systematic review. *JAMA*. 2003;289:2849–2856.
18. Schiff GD, Hasan O, Seijeoung K, et al. Diagnostic error in medicine. Analysis of 583 physician-reported errors. *Arch Intern Med*. 2009;169:1881–1887.
19. Guly HR. Diagnostic errors in an accident and emergency department. *Emerg Med J*. 2001;18:263–269.
20. Kuperman GJ, Boyle D, Jha A, et al. How promptly are inpatients treated for critical laboratory results? *J Am Med Inform Assoc*. 1998;5:112–119.
21. Borgstede JP, Lewis RS, Bhargavan M, Sunshine JH. RADPEER quality assurance program: a multifacility study of interpretive disagreement rates. *J Am Coll Radiol*. 2004;1:59–65.
22. Raab SS, Grzybicki DM, Janosky JE, et al. Clinical impact and frequency of anatomic pathology errors in cancer diagnoses. *Cancer*. 2005;104:2205–2213.
23. Lester JF, Dojcinov SD, Attanoos RL, et al. The clinical impact of expert pathological review on lymphoma management: a regional experience, *Br J Haematol*. 2003;123:463–468.
24. Croskerry P. Clinical cognition and diagnostic error: applications of a dual process model of reasoning. *Adv Health Sci Educ Theory Pract*. 2009;14:27–35.

25. Elstein AS. Thinking about diagnostic thinking: a 30-year perspective. *Adv Health Sci Educ Theory Pract*. 2009;14:7–18.
26. Eva KW. What every teacher needs to know about clinical reasoning. *Med Educ*. 2004;39:98–106.
27. Ark T, Brooks LR, Eva KW. The benefits of flexibility: the pedagogical value of instructions to adopt multifaceted diagnostic reasoning strategies. *Med Educ*. 2007;41:281–287.
28. Masicampo EJ, Baumeister RF. Toward a physiology of dual-process reasoning and judgment lemonade, willpower, and expensive rule-based analysis. *Psychol Sci*. 2008;19:255–260.
29. Friedman CP, Gatti GG, Franz TM, et al. Do physicians know when their diagnoses are correct? Implications for decision support and error reduction. *J Gen Intern Med*. 2005;20:334–339.
30. Elstein AS, Shulman LS, Sprafka SA. *Medical problem solving: an analysis of clinical reasoning*. Cambridge, MA: Harvard University Press; 1978:vii–xi.
31. Norman G. Building on experience—the development of clinical reasoning *N Engl J Med*. 2006;355:2251–2252.
32. Norman GR, Rosenthal D, Brooks LR, Allen SW, Muzzin LJ. The development of expertise in dermatology. *Arch Dermatol*. 1989;125:1063–1068.
33. Groves M, O'Rourke P, Alexander H. The clinical reasoning characteristics of diagnostic experts. *Med Teach*. 2003;25:308–313.
34. Croskerry P, Norman G. Overconfidence in clinical decision making. *Am J Med*. 2008;121(5A):S24–S29.
35. Klein JG. Five pitfalls in decisions about diagnosis and prescribing. *BMJ*. 2005;330:781–784.
36. Norman G. Dual processing and diagnostic errors. *Adv Health Sci Educ Theory Pract*. 2009;14:37–49.
37. Croskerry P. The Importance of cognitive errors in diagnosis and strategies to minimize them. *Acad Med*. 2003;78:775–780.
38. Redelmeier DA. The cognitive psychology of missed diagnoses. *Ann Intern Med*. 2005;142:115–120.
39. Kulatunga-Moruzi C, Brooks LR, Norman GR. Using comprehensive feature lists to bias medical diagnosis. *J Exp Psychol Learn Mem Cogn*. 2004;30:563–572.
40. Kern L, Doherty ME. 'Pseudodiagnosticity' in an idealized medical problem solving environment. *J Med Educ*. 1982;57:100–104.
41. Redelmeier DA, Shafir E, Aujla PS. The beguiling pursuit of more information. *Med Decis Making*. 2001;21:376–381.
42. Redelmeier DA, Tversky A. On the belief that arthritis pain is related to the weather. *Proc Natl Acad Sci USA*. 1996;93;2895–2896.
43. Redelmeier DA, Shafir E. Medical decision making in situations that offer multiple alternatives. *JAMA*. 1995;273:302–305
44. McNeil BJ, Pauker SG, Sox HC Jr., Tversky A. On the elicitation of preferences for alternative therapies. *N Engl J Med*. 1982;306:1259–1262.
45. Eva KW, Link CL, Lutfey KE, McKinlay JB. Swapping horses midstream: factors related to physicians' changing their minds about a diagnosis. *Acad Med*. 2010;85:1112–1117.
46. Miniati M, Monti S, Bottai M. A structured clinical model for predicting the probability of pulmonary embolism. *Am J Med*. 2003;114:173–179.
47. Hatala R, Norman GR, Brooks LR. Influence of a single example upon subsequent electrocardiogram interpretation. *Teach Learn Med*. 1999;11:110–117.
48. National Patient Safety Foundation. Available at: http://www.npsf.org/hp/psaw/download/A-Checklist-for-Getting-the-Right-Diagnosis-Working-with-Your-Doctor-or-Nurse.doc. Accessed April 5, 2010.
49. Simel DL, Rennie D. *The rational clinical examination. Evidence-based clinical diagnosis*. New York: McGraw Hill Medical; 2009.
50. Kassirer J. Diagnostic reasoning. *Ann Int Med*. 1989;110:893–900.
51. Rudolph JW, Morrison JB. Sidestepping superstitious learning, ambiguity, and other roadblocks: a feedback model of diagnostic problem solving. *Am J Med*. 2008;121(5A):S34–S37.
52. Schiff GD, Bates DW. Can electronic clinical documentation help prevent diagnostic errors? *N Engl J Med*. 2010;362:1066–1069.
53. Farnan JM, Johnson JK, Meltzer DO, Humphrey HJ, Arora VM. Resident uncertainty in clinical decision making and impact on patient care: a qualitative study. *Qual Saf Health Care*. 2008;17:122–126.
54. Pronovost P, Needham D, Berenholtz S, et al. An intervention to decrease catheter-related bloodstream infections in the ICU. *N Engl J Med*. 2006;355:2725–2732.
55. Kassirer JP. A report card on computer-assisted diagnosis—the grade: C. *N Engl J Med*. 1994;330:1824–1825.
56. Berner ES, Webster GD, Shugerman AA et al. Performance of four computer-based diagnostic systems. *N Engl J Med*. 1994;330:1792–1796.
57. Graber ML, Mathew A. Performance of a web-based clinical diagnosis support system for internists. *J Gen Intern Med*. 2008;23Suppl 1:37–40.

58. Valenstein PN. Formatting pathology reports applying four design principles to improve communication and patient safety. *Arch Pathol Lab Med*. 2008;132:84–94.
59. Wagar EA, Stankovic AK, Wilkinson DS, Walsh M, Souers RJ. Assessment monitoring of laboratory critical values: a College of American Pathologists Q-Tracks study of 180 institutions. *Arch Pathol Lab Med*. 2007;131:44–49.
60. Joanne C, Andrew G, Julie L, Johanna IW. The safety implications of missed test results for hospitalised patients: a systematic review. *BMJ Qual Saf*. 2010. 10.1136/bmjqs.2010.044339. Accessed February 15, 2011.
61. Singh H, Arora HS, Vij MS, Raghuram R, Khan MM, Petersen LA. Communication outcomes of critical imaging results in a computerized notification system. *J Am Med Inform Assoc*. 2007;14:459–466.
62. Patal AK, Poon EG, Karson AS, Gandhi TK, Roy CL. Lessons learned from implementation of a computerized application for pending tests at hospital discharge. *J Hosp Med*. 2011;6:16–21.

CHAPTER 3

CRACKING THE CASE

JENNEI WEI
Department of Medicine, University of California, San Francisco, California

PATRICK P. KNEELAND
Division of Hospital Medicine, Providence Regional Medical Center, Everett, Washington

GURPREET DHALIWAL
Department of Medicine, University of California, San Francisco, California; Medical Service, San Francisco VA Medical Center, San Francisco, California

A 43-year-old woman presented to an outside hospital with painful plaques and patches on her bilateral lower extremities. Two weeks prior to this presentation, she had noticed a single red lesion on her left ankle. Over the next 2 weeks, the lesion enlarged to involve the lower half of her posterior calf and subsequently turned purple and became exquisitely tender. Similar but smaller purple, tender lesions simultaneously appeared, first over her right shin and then on her bilateral thighs and hips. She also reported fatigue as well as diffuse joint pains in her hands and wrists bilaterally for the past month. She denied any swelling of these joints or functional impairment. She denied fevers, weight loss, headache, sinus symptoms, difficulty breathing, or abdominal pain.

Although we do not yet have a physical exam, the tempo, pattern of spread, and accompanying features allow some early hypotheses to be considered. Distal lower extremity lesions that darkened and spread could be erythema nodosum or erythema induratum. Malignancies rarely have such prominent skin manifestations, although leukemia cutis or an aggressive cutaneous T-cell lymphoma might present with disseminated and darkened plaques, and Kaposi's sarcoma is characteristically purple and multifocal. Autoimmune disorders such as sarcoidosis, cutaneous lupus, and psoriasis may similarly present with widespread plaques. Most disseminated infections that start with patches evolve to pustules, ulcers, bullae, or other forms that reflect the invasive nature of the infection; syphilis warrants consideration for any widespread eruption of unknown etiology. Antecedent arthralgias with fatigue suggest an autoimmune condition, although infections such as hepatitis or parvovirus can do the same. Systemic lupus erythematosus (SLE) or rheumatoid arthritis (RA) would be favored initially on account of her demographics and the hand and wrist involvement, and each can be associated with vasculitis.

Clinical Care Conundrums: Challenging Diagnoses in Hospital Medicine, First Edition.
Edited by James C. Pile, Thomas E. Baudendistel, and Brian J. Harte.

The significant pain as described is not compatible with most of the aforementioned diagnoses. Its presence, coupled with potential autoimmune symptoms, suggests a vasculitis such as polyarteritis nodosa (which can have prominent diffuse skin involvement), Henoch Schonlein purpura (with its predilection for the lower extremities, including extension to the hips and buttocks), cryoglobulinemia, or SLE- or RA-associated vasculitis. Calciphylaxis is another ischemic vascular disorder that can cause diffuse dark painful lesions, but this only warrants consideration if advanced renal disease is present.

A skin biopsy of her right hip was taken at an outside hospital. She was discharged on a 2-week course of prednisone for suspected vasculitis while biopsy results were pending. Over the next 2 weeks, none of the skin lesions improved, despite compliance with this treatment, and the skin over her left posterior calf and right shin lesions began to erode and bleed. In addition, small purple tender lesions appeared over the pinnae of both ears. Three weeks after her initial evaluation, she presented to another emergency department for ulcerating skin lesions and worsening pain. At that point, the initial skin biopsy result was available and revealed "vasculopathy of the small vessels with thrombi but no vasculitis."

The patient had no children and denied a history of miscarriages. Her past medical history was unremarkable. She did not report any history of thrombotic events. She started a new job as a software engineer 1 month ago and was feeling stressed about her new responsibilities. She denied any high-risk sexual behavior and any history of intravenous drug use. She had not traveled recently and did not own any pets. There was no family history of rheumatologic disorders, hypercoagulable states, or thrombotic events.

This picture of occluded but noninflamed vessels shifts the diagnosis away from vasculitis and focuses attention on hypercoagulable states with prominent dermal manifestations, including antiphospholipid antibody syndrome (APLS) and livedoid vasculopathy. In this young woman with arthralgias, consideration of SLE and APLS is warranted. Her recent increase in stress and widespread purpuric and ulcerative lesions could bring to mind a factitious disorder, but the histology results eliminate this possibility.

The patient's temperature was 36.5°C, her blood pressure was 110/70 mm Hg, respiratory rate was 16 breaths per minute, and her heart rate was 65 beats per minute. She was well-appearing but in moderate pain. She did not have any oral lesions. Her cardiac, respiratory, and abdominal exams were normal. Skin exam revealed a 10-cm by 4-cm area of bloody granulation tissue draining serosanguinous fluid, surrounded by stellate palpable netlike purpura on her left posterior calf. There was a similar 4-cm by 2-cm ulcerated lesion on her right shin. Both lesions were exquisitely tender to palpation. On her bilateral thighs and hips, there were multiple stellate purpuric patches, all 4 cm in diameter or less, and only minimally tender to palpation. She also had 1-cm purpuric bullae on the helices of both ears (Fig. 3.1), which were slightly tender to palpation. Splinter hemorrhages were also noted on multiple nail beds bilaterally. Musculoskeletal exam did not reveal any synovitis.

The original purpura on her calf and ear demonstrate a clear demarcation corresponding to cutaneous vascular insufficiency. The development of bullae (ear) and ulceration (calf) are compatible with ischemia. Despite the presence of multiple splinter hemorrhages, the distribution of lesions is very unusual for an embolic phenomenon (eg, endocarditis, cholesterol emboli, or atrial myxoma). The multifocal nature of the skin

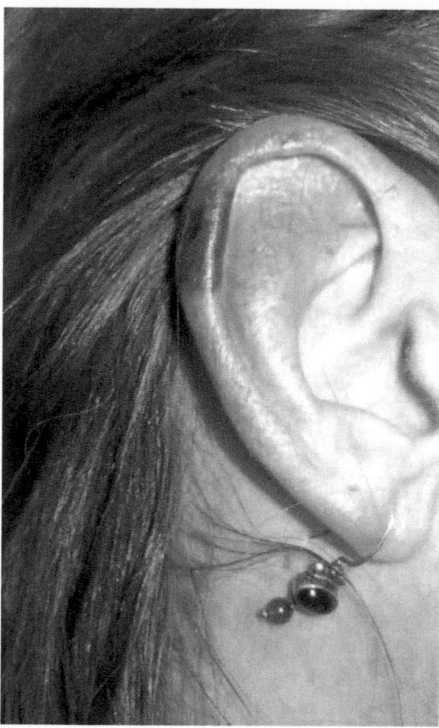

FIGURE 3.1 Purpuric bullous lesion involving the ear.

lesions with progression to well-demarcated cutaneous necrosis is reminiscent of calciphylaxis or warfarin-induced skin necrosis, although she lacks the relevant risk factors. A toxin such as cocaine or methamphetamine mediating multifocal vasoconstriction or hypercoagulability should be excluded.

The bilateral ear involvement remains decidedly unusual and makes me wonder if there is something about the ear, such as the nature of its circulation or its potentially lower temperature (as an acral organ) that might render it particularly susceptible, for instance, to cryoglobulinemia or cryofibrinogenemia-mediated ischemia.

Laboratory studies demonstrated the following: white blood cell count, 1500/mm^3 (37.3% neutrophils, 5.1% lymphocytes, 6.7% monocytes, and 1.3% eosinophils); hemoglobin, 9.3 g/dL (mean corpuscular volume, 91 fL); platelet count, 212/mm^3; erythrocyte sedimentation rate, 62 mm/hour; and C-reactive protein, 14.6 mg/L. Serum electrolytes, liver tests, coagulation studies, and urinalysis were normal. Fecal occult blood test was negative.

The patient's neutropenia and anemia suggest decreased production in the marrow by infection, malignancy, or toxin, or increased destruction, perhaps from an autoimmune process. The associated infections are usually viral, such as human immunodeficiency virus (HIV) and Epstein-Barr virus (EBV), although their linkage with the cutaneous disease in the patient is tenuous. It is possible that malignancy could be present in the marrow with resultant dermal hypercoagulability and ischemia, but this seems unlikely. We do not know about any toxins that she has been exposed to, but these hematologic findings would mandate directed inquiry along those lines. In this young woman with cutaneous ulcers secondary to thrombotic vasculopathy, bicytopenia, antecedent arthralgias without synovitis, and elevated inflammatory markers, I favor an autoimmune process such as SLE, which I would evaluate with an antinuclear antibody (ANA) and antiphospholipid antibody studies.

She was admitted to the hospital and received hydromorphone for pain control. Corticosteroids were not administered. Peripheral blood morphology was normal. Antibodies against HIV1 and 2 were negative, as were antibodies against cytomegalovirus, EBV, parvovirus B19, *Mycoplasma pneumoniae*, and hepatitis C virus. Bilateral lower-extremity ultrasound was negative for deep vein thrombosis. Transthoracic echocardiogram was normal. Repeat skin biopsy confirmed small vessel vasculopathy without vasculitis (Fig. 3.2). The results of the following investigations were also negative: ANA, rheumatoid factor, double-stranded DNA (dsDNA), cyclic citrullinated peptide, ribonucleoprotein (RNP), and anti-Smith antibodies. C3 and C4 complement levels were normal.

Given how much the histology is driving the clinical reasoning and focusing the differential diagnosis in this case, I agree with the decision to repeat the biopsy. In complex or undiagnosed cases, repeat histology samples allow for confirmation of the original interpretation (often with the perspective of new clinicians and pathologists) and sometimes reveal pathognomonic or additional findings that appear only after the disease has evolved over time. HIV seronegativity helps constrain the differential diagnosis, and parvovirus is another excellent consideration for arthralgias and cytopenias (with the predilection to involve cell lines other than RBCs particularly seen in HIV), although ulcers are not seen with this condition. Herpes simplex virus (HSV) is another viral infection that can cause painful skin ulcerations and cytopenias, although the duration and distribution are highly atypical. The negative ANA and dsDNA and normal complement levels make SLE unlikely. The negative lower extremity ultrasound helps frame the thromboses as a local cutaneous process rather than a systemic hypercoagulable state. Although the peripheral blood smear is normal, a bone marrow biopsy will be necessary to exclude a marrow invasive process, such as leukemia or lymphoma. A bone marrow biopsy would also provide another opportunity to examine tissue for mycobacteria or fungi, which can cause ulcerations and cytopenias, although there is little reason to suspect she is susceptible to those pathogens. As this clinical picture fails to fit clearly with an infectious, autoimmune, or neoplastic disorder, I would revisit the possibility

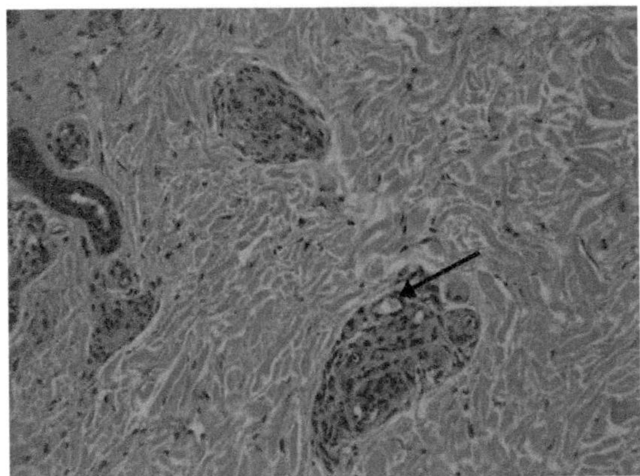

FIGURE 3.2 Punch biopsy of left calf lesion revealing blood vessel occluded by fibrin thrombi (arrow).

of toxins—prescription, complementary, over-the-counter, or illegal (eg, cocaine) at this time.

In further discussion with the patient, she reported using cocaine intranasally for the past 3 months. Her urine toxicology was positive for cocaine. She was found to have positive perinuclear antineutrophil cytoplasmic antibodies (p-ANCAs), antimyeloperoxidase (MPO) antibodies, anticardiolipin (ACL) antibodies, and lupus anticoagulant (LAC). By hospital day 3, her lesions had significantly improved without any intervention and her absolute neutrophil count increased to 1080/mm^3.

The presence of widespread cutaneous ischemia (with bland thrombosis) and detectable ACL and LAC antibodies is compatible with APLS; the APLS could be deemed primary because there is no clear associated rheumatologic or any other systemic disease. However, neutropenia is not a characteristic of APLS, which has thrombocytopenia as its more frequently associated hematologic abnormality. Livedoid vasculopathy, a related disorder, is also supported by the ACL and LAC results, but also does not feature neutropenia. While the presence of diffuse thrombosis could be attributed to a widespread secondary effect of cocaine vasoconstriction, the appearance of ANCA (which can be drug-induced, eg, propylthiouracil [PTU]) and the slowly resolving neutropenia during hospitalization without specific treatment is very suggestive of a toxin. The demographic diffuse skin ulcers and hematologic and serologic profile are compatible with the recently described toxidrome related to levamisole adulteration of cocaine.

A sendout study of a urine sample returned positive for levamisole. Based on purpuric skin lesions with a predilection for the ears, agranulocytosis, and skin biopsy revealing thrombotic vasculopathy, she was diagnosed with levamisole-adulterated cocaine exposure. One week after discharge, her lower extremity pain and ulcerations significantly improved. Her absolute neutrophil count increased to 2820/mm^3. Her urine toxicology screen was negative for cocaine.

DISCUSSION

Levamisole was initially developed in 1964 as an antihelminthic agent. Its incidentally discovered immunomodulatory effects led to trials for the treatment of chronic infections, inflammatory bowel disease, rheumatic diseases,[1] and nephrotic syndrome in children.[2] By 1990, three major studies supported levamisole as an adjunctive therapy in melanoma[3] and colon cancer.[4]

Although levamisole appeared to be nontoxic at single or low doses, long-term use in clinical trials demonstrated that 2.5%-13% of patients developed life-threatening agranulocytosis, and up to 10% of those instances resulted in death.[5] A distinctive cutaneous pseudovasculitis was noted in children on therapeutic levamisole. They presented with purpura that had a predilection for the ears, cheeks, and thighs[6] and positive serologic markers for ANCA and antiphospholipid antibodies. Skin biopsies of the purpuric lesions revealed leukocytoclastic vasculitis, thrombotic vasculitis, and/or vascular occlusions.

Levamisole was withdrawn from the market in 2000 in the United States due to its side effects,[7] but it quickly found its way onto the black market. It was first detected in cocaine in 2002, and since then, the percentage of cocaine containing levamisole has steadily been increasing. In July 2009, over 70% of cocaine seized by the Drug Enforcement Administration was found to contain levamisole.[8] It is unclear exactly why this drug is used as an adulterant in cocaine. Theories include potentiation of the euphoric effects of cocaine, serving as a bulking agent, or functioning as a chemical signature to track distribution.[9]

The resurgence of levamisole has brought a new face to a problem that occurred over a decade ago. Current reports of levamisole toxicity describe adults presenting with purpura preferentially involving the ears, neutropenia, positive ANCA, and positive antiphospholipid antibodies.[10–12] Since 2002, there have been at least 20 confirmed cases of agranulocytosis and two deaths associated with levamisole-adulterated cocaine.[8,13,14] In September 2009, the Department of Health and Human Services issued a public health alert warning of an impending increase in levamisole-related illness.

Levamisole is not detected in routine toxicology screens, but can be tested for using gas chromatography and mass spectrometry. Most laboratories do not offer testing for levamisole and sendout testing is required. Given its half-life of 5.6 hours, levamisole can only be detected in the blood within 24 hours and in the urine within 48–72 hours of exposure.[15,16] Urine samples are preferred over blood samples because blood levels decline more rapidly and have lower sensitivity. Cocaine samples can also be sent out to local or state forensics laboratories to be tested for levamisole. The only definitive treatment for levamisole-induced cutaneous pseudovasculitis and neutropenia is cessation of toxin exposure.

Although the discussant was familiar with this toxidrome from local and published cases, he was only able to settle on levamisole toxicity after a series of competing hypotheses were ruled out on the basis of irreconcilable features (vasculitis and histology results; APLS and neutropenia; SLE and negative ANA with no visceral involvement) and by using analogical reasoning (e.g., to infer the presence of a toxin on the basis of neutropenia [as seen with chemotherapy and other drugs] and ANCA induction [as seen with PTU]). It was a laborious process of hypothesis testing, but one that ultimately allowed him to crack the case.

Key Points

1. In patients presenting with neutropenia and purpuric skin lesions—particularly with a predilection for the ears—consider levamisole-adulterated cocaine exposure.
2. Tests supporting this diagnosis include positive serologies for ANCA and antiphospholipid antibodies and skin biopsies that show leukocytoclastic vasculitis, thrombotic vasculitis, or vascular occlusion. Urine studies for levamisole are definitive if sent within 48–72 hours of exposure.

This case was presented by the authors (JW, PPK) at the Society of Hospital Medicine Annual Meeting in April 2010. This case was also described briefly (two paragraphs with images) in a research letter in the March 2010 issue of the *Journal of the American Academy of Dermatology*.[12]

REFERENCES

1. Amery WK, Bruynseels JP. Levamisole, the story and the lessons. *Int J Immunopharmocol*. 1992; 14(3):481–486.
2. British Association for Paediatric Nephrology. Levamisole for corticosteroid-dependent nephrotic syndrome in childhood. *Lancet*. 1991;337:1555–1557.
3. Quirt I, Shelley W, Pater J, Bodurtha A, McCulloch P. Improved survival in patients with poor-prognosis malignant melanoma treated with adjuvant levamisole: A phase III study by the National Cancer Institute of Canada Clinical Trials Group. *J Clin Oncol*. 1991;9:729–735.

4. Moertel CG, Fleming TR, MacDonald JS. Levamisole and fluorouracil for adjuvant therapy of resected colon carcinoma. *N Engl J Med*. 1990;322:352–358.
5. Thompson JS, Herbick JM, Klassen LW. Studies on levamisole-induced agranulocytosis. *Blood*. 1980;56(3):388–396.
6. Rongioletti F, Ghio L, Ginevri F. Purpura of the ears: A distinctive vasculopathy with circulating autoantibodies complicating long-term treatment with levamisole in children. *Br J Dermatol*. 1999;140:948–951.
7. Frederick J. Janssen discontinues ergamisol. Available at: http://findarticles.com/p/articles/mi_m3374/is_18_22/ai_68536218/. Accessed July 25, 2010.
8. SAMHSA. Nationwide public health alert issued concerning life-threatening risk posed by cocaine laced with veterinary anti-parasite drug. Available at: http://www.samhsa.gov/newsroom/advisories/090921vet5101.aspx. Accessed July 20, 2010.
9. Fucci N. Unusual adulterants in cocaine seized on Italian clandestine market. *Forensic Sci Int*. 2007;172(2–3):e1.
10. Buchanan JA, Vogel JA, Eberhardt AM. Levamisole-induced occlusive necrotizing vasculitis of the ears after use of cocaine contaminated with levamisole. *J Med Toxicol*. 2011;7(1):83–84.
11. Bradford M, Rosenberg B, Moreno J, Dumyati G. Bilateral necrosis of earlobes and cheeks: another complication of cocaine contaminated with levamisole. *Ann Intern Med*. 2010;152(11):758–759.
12. Waller JM, Feramisco JD, Alberta-Wszolek L, McCalmont TH, Fox LP. Cocaine-associated retiform purpura and neutropenia: is levamisole the culprit? *J Am Acad Dermatol*. 2010;63(3):530–535.
13. Buchanan JA, Oyer RJ, Patel NR, Jacquet GA. A confirmed case of agranulocytosis after use of cocaine contaminated with levamisole. *J Med Toxicol*. 2010;6(2):160–164.
14. Centers for Disease Control and Prevention. Agranulocytosis associated with cocaine use—four States, March 2008–November 2009. *MMWR*. 2009;58(49):1381–1385.
15. Morley SR, Forrest AR, Galloway JH. Levamisole as a contaminant of illicit cocaine. *Journal of the Clandestine Laboratory Investigating Chemists Association*. 2006;16:6–11. Available at: http://www.tiaft2006.org/proceedings/pdf/PT-p-06.pdf. Accessed July 20, 2010.
16. LeGatt DF. Cocaine cutting agents—a discussion. Laboratory Medicine and Pathology, University of Alberta. Available at: http://www.vandu.org/documents/Levamisole_Cocaine.pdf. Accessed July 20, 2010.

CHAPTER 4

A MIDLIFE CRISIS

JENNIFER R. LUKELA and RAJESH S. MANGRULKAR
Department of Internal Medicine, University of Michigan, Ann Arbor, Michigan

LAWRENCE M. TIERNEY JR.
Department of Medicine, University of California, San Francisco, California

JOHN DEL VALLE
Department of Internal Medicine, University of Michigan, Ann Arbor, Michigan

SANJAY SAINT
Department of Internal Medicine, University of Michigan, Ann Arbor, Michigan; Ann Arbor VA Health Services Research and Development Field Program, Ann Arbor, Michigan; Patient Safety Enhancement Program, University of Michigan Health System, Ann Arbor, Michigan; Tuscan-American Safety Collaborative, Florence, Italy

A 47-year-old woman was brought to the emergency department by her family because of 1 week of abdominal pain. The pain had begun in the epigastrium but had spread across the abdomen. She described it as constant and 10 of 10 in intensity but could not identify aggravating or alleviating factors. She also complained of nausea and vomiting, beginning 4 days prior to presentation, occurring two to five times per day. She noted poor oral intake and mild diarrhea. She denied melena or hematochezia. She reported no recent fever, dysuria, chills, or night sweats; however, she reported upper respiratory symptoms 2 weeks prior to presentation. On the day of presentation, her family felt she was becoming increasingly lethargic.

Epigastric pain in a middle-aged woman suggests several possible diagnoses. Conditions such as acute cholecystitis begin abruptly, whereas small bowel obstruction, appendicitis, and diverticulitis start gradually. Nausea and vomiting are common concomitants of abdominal pain and are nonspecific. The absence of fever and chills is reassuring. Of greatest concern is the patient's mental status. Initially, I think of enterohemorrhagic *Escherichia coli* syndromes with associated glomerulonephritis.

The patient had a history of nephrolithiasis and had undergone total abdominal hysterectomy and bilateral salpingo-oopherectomy secondary to uterine fibroids. She took occasional acetaminophen, smoked two cigarettes per day, and rarely consumed alcohol. Temperature was 38.5°C, heart rate was 160 beats per minute, respiratory rate was 28/minute, and blood pressure was 92/52 mm Hg; oxygen saturation was 100% breathing 2 L of oxygen by nasal cannula. She was a moderately obese African-American woman in moderate distress, lying in bed moaning. Mucous membranes were dry. There was no lymphadenopathy or thyromegaly.

Clinical Care Conundrums: Challenging Diagnoses in Hospital Medicine, First Edition.
Edited by James C. Pile, Thomas E. Baudendistel, and Brian J. Harte.

Heart rate was regular without appreciable murmur, rub, or gallop. Lungs were clear. Abdomen was soft and nondistended, with diffuse tenderness to palpation; bowel sounds were present; there was no rebound or guarding. She had normal rectal tone with brown, guaiac-negative stool. There was no costovertebral angle tenderness. She was oriented to person, place, and time but lethargic; deep tendon reflexes were 3+ bilaterally, and no focal neurologic signs were elicited.

Renal stones certainly produce abdominal pain, and the rare patient undergoes laparotomy for this reason. The hysterectomy tells us that small bowel obstruction could be a reason for her symptoms, although abnormal mental status would not be expected without additional problems such as infection. The tachycardia seems out of proportion to her temperature. Hyperpnea and absent respiratory symptoms, along with hypotension and tachycardia, suggest a sepsis syndrome. Her physical exam confirms dehydration. Examination of the abdomen makes me speculate about whether she has a nonsurgical cause of acute abdomen. The lethargy remains unexplained. Sepsis syndrome, possibly from a perinephric abscess, is my leading diagnosis.

White blood cell count was 15.9/mm^3 with 78% neutrophils, hemoglobin was 14.3 g/dL with an MCV of 76 and a platelet count of 320/mm^3. Sodium was 159 mmol/L; chloride, 128 mmol/L; bicarbonate, 19 mmol/L; blood urea nitrogen, 120 mmol/L; creatinine 3.1, mg/dL; calcium, 11.7 mg/dL; albumin, 3.3 g/dL; serum aspartate aminotransferase, 65 U/L; serum alanine aminotransferase, 72 U/L; total bilirubin, 0.7 mg/dL; amylase, 137 U/L (normal 30–100); and lipase, 92 IU/dL (normal 4–24). Urine obtained from Foley catheter revealed negative nitrite and leukocyte esterase, 50–75 red blood cells, and 10–25 white blood cells per high-powered field.

The elevated serum sodium is likely contributing to her abnormal mental status. It is unusual for a previously healthy and conscious woman to become this hypernatremic because persons with a normal mental status will defend their sodium balance strenuously, assuming regulatory mechanisms are intact. Generally, this level of hypernatremia indicates two things: one, a patient was not allowed, or did not seek access to, free water and the other is the presence of diabetes insipidus. It is unlikely she became this dehydrated from the initial gastrointestinal episode as described. The low MCV suggests she may be a thalassemia carrier, as microcytosis with iron deficiency typically does not occur until the patient is anemic, although she may be when rehydrated. Serum calcium, while elevated, also will likely return to the normal range with hydration. The metabolic abnormalities strongly suggest a problem in the central nervous system. The hematuria in the urinalysis continues to raise the possibility of nephrolithiasis as a cause of abdominal pain, although it does not fit well with the rest of the patient's clinical picture. The hematuria and pyuria both could still indicate a urinary tract infection such as pyelonephritis or perinephric abscess causing a sepsis syndrome.

An acute abdominal series and chest radiograph revealed a paucity of gas in the abdomen but no free air under the diaphragm or active cardiopulmonary disease. Abdominal ultrasound showed cholelithiasis without biliary dilation. There was no evidence of hydronephrosis, hydroureter, or perinephric abscess. A noncontrast abdominal-pelvic computed tomography (CT) **scan demonstrated no peripancreatic stranding or fluid collection and no nephrolithiasis or fluid collection suggestive of abscess. The admission electrocardiogram, read as sinus tachycardia with a rate of 160, is displayed in Fig. 4.1.**

I have long believed that unexplained sinus tachycardia is one of the most ominous rhythms in clinical medicine; it is expected after vigorous exercise, among other

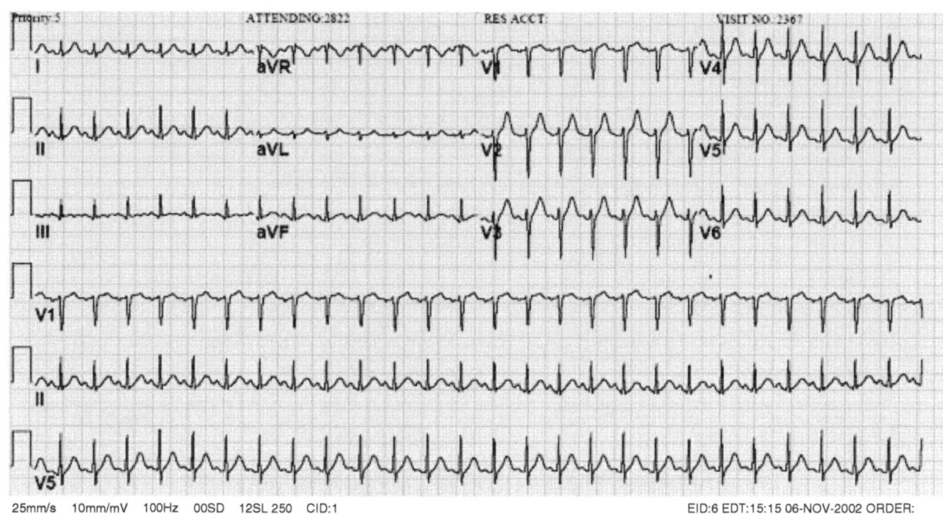

FIGURE 4.1 Electrocardiogram obtained at the time of admission. Interpreted as sinus tachycardia at a rate of 160 with a short PR interval.

situations, but not in the condition in which this woman finds herself. The nature of the tracing does not indicate the likelihood of a supraventricular arrhythmia, particularly atrial flutter, which should be considered given the rate. The absence of free air under the diaphragm on chest radiography is reassuring. Although the pancreatic enzymes are mildly elevated, they are usually far more striking in gallstone pancreatitis. Hypercalcemia may result in abdominal pain by several mechanisms. I remain concerned about her central nervous system.

The patient was admitted to the intensive care unit (ICU)**, where she received intravenous antibiotics and aggressive rehydration. The following morning she continued to complain of abdominal pain. Her systolic blood pressure was 115 mm Hg, and her heart rate ranged between 140 and 150 beats per minute. The remainder of her physical exam was unchanged. Repeat laboratory tests revealed a white blood cell count of 14.7/mm^3, a blood urea nitrogen of 66 mg/dL, a creatinine of 1.3 mg/dL, an amylase of 67 IU/L, and a lipase of 70 IU/dL. A contrast-enhanced abdominal-pelvic CT scan did not reveal intra-abdominal pathology. Blood and urine cultures obtained at admission were negative for any growth.**

The patient was appropriately admitted to the ICU. When caring for a critically ill patient, establishing a diagnosis is less important initially than addressing treatable conditions with dispatch. The negative CT scans rule out previously entertained diagnoses such as nephrolithiasis and perinephric abscess. It is possible that the initially positive urinalysis was a result of urinary catheter placement trauma. Given the course to date, I believe this patient likely has a nonsurgical cause of abdominal pain. I am considering entities such as lead intoxication, hypercalcemia, tear of the rectus abdominus caused by vomiting, systemic vasculitis, or a hypercoagulable state leading to intra-abdominal venous thrombosis.

By hospital day 3, her sodium decreased to 149 mmol/L and her creatinine was 1.0 mg/dL. Abdominal pain persisted, unchanged from admission. Her systolic blood pressure had stabilized at 120 mm Hg, but the heart rate remained near 150 beats per minute. Her abdomen remained soft and nondistended on exam but

diffusely tender to palpation. Her amylase and lipase continued to decrease, and her repeat electrocardiogram demonstrated tachycardia with a rate of 144.

We are gratified to see that her serum sodium has waned but not with the persistence of the tachycardia. It must be assumed that this patient has an infectious disease that we are not clever enough to diagnose at this time. I am also considering an autoimmune process, such as systemic lupus erythematosus. It is difficult to envision a neoplastic disorder causing these problems. The differential remains broad, however, because we have not ruled out metabolic or endocrine causes. It is difficult to imagine she could have Addison's disease—a common cause of severe abdominal pain, tachycardia, and hypotension—given her serum sodium level. Hyperthyroidism has been known to produce mild hypercalcemia and abdominal complaints and is an intriguing possibility. The striking elevation of her serum sodium makes me consider the possibility of a problem in the posterior pituitary gland, such as sarcoidosis. I cannot explain how sarcoidosis would cause her abdominal pain, unless the hypercalcemia were related. The tachycardia remains of concern, especially if she is otherwise improving. Thus, I would likely administer a small dose of adenosine to ascertain that this is not a different supraventricular tachycardia. In sinus tachycardia, the rate is usually attendant to the clinical picture and thus begs explanation given her clinical improvement.

After receiving 6 mg of intravenous adenosine, the patient's heart rate declined; atrial flutter waves were observed.

This case nicely demonstrates a key teaching point: a fast regular heart rate of about 150, irrespective of the electrocardiogram, suggests atrial flutter. Who gets atrial flutter? Patients with chronic lung disease, myocardial ischemia (albeit rarely), alcohol-induced cardiomyopathy, and infiltrative cardiac disorders. Additionally, we also have to consider thyroid dysfunction.

If forced to come up with a single unifying diagnosis at this point, I would have to say this patient most likely has sarcoidosis because this entity would account for modest hypercalcemia, the myocardial conduction disturbance, and hypernatremia because of diabetes insipidus; furthermore, it would fit the patient's demographic profile. However, I am also concerned about hyperthyroidism and would not proceed until thyroid function studies were obtained.

Thyroid studies revealed thyroid stimulating hormone of less than 0.01 mU/L (normal range, 0.30–5.50), free thyroxine (T4) of 5.81 ng/dL (normal range, 0.73–1.79), free triiodothyronine (T3) of 15.7 pg/mL (normal range, 2.8–5.3), and total triiodothyronine (T3) of 218 ng/dL (normal range, 95–170). The patient was diagnosed with thyroid crisis and was started on propranolol, propylthiouracil, hydrocortisone, and a saturated solution of potassium iodine. Thyroid stimulating immunoglobulins were obtained and found to be markedly elevated (3.4 TSI index; normal < 1.3), suggestive of Grave's disease. Over the next several days, the patient's abdominal pain and tachycardia resolved. Her mental status returned to normal. A workup for her microcytosis anemia revealed beta-thalassemia trait. The patient was discharged home on hospital day 9 and has done well as an outpatient.

COMMENTARY

As Sir Zachary Cope stated in his classic text *Cope's Early Diagnosis of the Acute Abdomen*, "It is only by thorough history taking and physical examination that one can propound a diagnosis."[1] When first presented with a patient whose chief complaint is abdominal pain, physicians tend to focus on the disorders of both the hollow and solid organs of the abdomen as potential sources of the pain. The differential diagnosis traditionally includes disorders such as cholecystitis, peptic ulcer disease, pancreatitis, small bowel obstruction, bowel ischemia or perforation, splenic abscess and infarct, nephrolithiasis, diverticulitis, and appendicitis, all of which were initially considered by the clinicians involved in this case. But as our discussant pointed out, in this case, the differential needed to be broadened to include less common disorders, particularly given the patient's altered mental status, numerous electrolyte abnormalities, and lethargy and the lack of explanation provided by the physical examination and sophisticated imaging studies.

Specifically, a myriad of systemic diseases and metabolic derangements can cause abdominal complaints *and* mimic surgical abdominal disease, including hypercalcemia, acute intermittent porphyria, diabetic ketoacidosis, lead intoxication, familial Mediterranean fever, vasculopathies, adrenal insufficiency, and hyperthyroidism. Unfortunately, the frequency with which abdominal pain occurs in many of these less common disease processes and the pathophysiology that underlies its occurrence are not well defined. For example, abdominal pain is well described as a typical manifestation of both diabetic ketoacidosis and lead poisoning, but the pathophysiology behind its occurrence is poorly understood in both. Furthermore, as a manifestation of thyrotoxicosis and as one of the diagnostic criteria for thyroid storm, the reported prevalence of abdominal pain in this condition is variable, ranging from "rare" to 20%–47%.[2–4] Also, although other gastrointestinal manifestations of hyperthyroidism (such as nausea, vomiting, and hyperdefecation) are thought to be the result of the effect of excess thyroid hormone on gastrointestinal motility, it is unclear whether this similar mechanism is responsible for the perception of abdominal pain.[4]

An important clue to the underlying diagnosis in this case was the patient's marked tachycardia. Classically, a persistent heart rate of 150 should raise suspicion of atrial flutter with a 2:1 conduction block, as was eventually discovered in this case. Adenosine, in addition to other vagal maneuvers such as carotid massage or Valsalva that also block atrioventricular (AV) node conduction, has been recognized as a safe and effective means of establishing a diagnosis in tachyarrhythmias.[5] In AV-node-dependent tachycardias, such as AV node reentrant tachycardia or AV reentrant tachycardia, adenosine will often terminate the tachyarrhythmia by blocking the anterograde limb of the reentrant circuit. In AV-node-independent tachyarrhythmias, such as atrial flutter or atrial fibrillation, adenosine will not terminate the rhythm. However, in the case of flutter, blocking the AV node will usually transiently unmask the underlying P waves, thereby facilitating the diagnosis.[5,6]

In this patient, the discovery of atrial flutter was the main clue that thyrotoxicosis may provide the unifying diagnosis. Thyroid hormone has a direct positive cardiac chronotropic effect, resulting in the increased resting heart characteristic of thyrotoxicosis. Specifically, this hormone increases sinoatrial node firing, shortens the refractory period of conduction tissue within the heart, and decreases the electrical threshold for atrial excitation. In addition to predisposing to sinus tachycardia (the most common rhythm associated with this disorder), thyrotoxicosis is also associated with atrial tachycardias such as atrial flutter and, more classically, atrial fibrillation.[7,8] Although no studies have specifically evaluated the incidence of atrial flutter in thyrotoxicosis, atrial fibrillation has been found in 9%–22% of these patients.[7]

Finally, several of the patient's electrolyte derangements could explain some of her clinical findings and are clues to the underlying diagnosis. She initially presented with a mild hypercalcemia that persisted even after hydration. Potential explanations include her severe dehydration or her underlying thyrotoxicosis because hypercalcemia is present in up to 20% of patients with hyperthyroidism.[9,10] However, the presence of significant hypercalcemia in the setting of thyrotoxicosis may actually make the diagnosis of thyrotoxicosis more difficult, masking the hypermetabolic signs and symptoms of the hyperthyroid state.[11] Interestingly, coexistent primary hyperparathyroidism does occur in a few of these patients, but it likely was not an underlying cause in our patient, given her calcium normalized after propylthiouracil therapy.[12]

The patient's marked hypernatremia is more difficult to explain. She may have developed nephrogenic diabetes insipidus secondary to hypercalcemia, explained by a renal concentrating defect that can become evident once the calcium is persistently above 11 mg/dL.[13] Combined with her altered mental status, which likely limited her ability to access free water, this may be enough to explain her marked hypernatremia. Her rapid improvement with rehydration is also consistent with this explanation, mediated through the improvement of her serum free calcium.

This case highlights the importance of using all the clinical clues provided by the history, physical exam, and laboratory and imaging studies when generating an initial differential diagnosis, as well as the importance of being willing to appropriately broaden and narrow the list of possibilities as a case evolves. When this patient was initially evaluated by physicians in the emergency department, they believed her symptoms were most consistent with generalized peritonitis that was likely secondary to an infectious or inflammatory intra-abdominal process such as pancreatitis (especially in light of her mildly elevated lipase and amylase), appendicitis, or diverticulitis. When the medical team in the ICU assumed care of this patient, members of the team failed to recognize several of the early clues, including the patient's markedly abnormal mental status, electrolyte derangements, and persistent tachycardia despite aggressive rehydration, which suggested the possibility of alternative, and less common, etiologies of her abdominal pain. Instead, they continued to aggressively pursue the possibility of the initial differential diagnosis, even repeating some of the previously negative studies from the emergency department. This case illustrates the importance of constantly reevaluating the available information from physical examination and laboratory and imaging studies and not falling victim to "intellectual blind spots" created by suggested diagnoses by other care providers. Fortunately, for this patient, her thyroid crisis was diagnosed, albeit with some delay, before any long-term complications occurred.

Key Points

1. A regular narrow-complex tachycardia of approximately 150 beats per minute should always prompt consideration of the possibility of atrial flutter.
2. A variety of "nonsurgical" conditions may cause diffuse abdominal pain and should be considered in the appropriate setting. These include thyrotoxicosis, hypercalcemia, acute intermittent porphyria, lead intoxication, familial Mediterranean fever, adrenal insufficiency, diabetic ketoacidosis, and vasculitis.

REFERENCES

1. Silen W, ed. *Cope's Early Diagnosis of the Acute Abdomen*. 19th ed. New York: Oxford University Press; 1995:4.
2. Harwood-Nuss AL, Martel TJ. An unusual cause of abdominal pain in young woman. *Ann Emerg Med*. 1991;20:574–582.

3. Harper MB. Vomiting, nausea and abdominal pain: unrecognized symptoms of thyrotoxicosis. *J Fam Prac*. 1989;24:382–386.
4. Powell DW, Alpers DH, Yamada T, Owyang C, Laine L, eds. *Textbook of Gastroenterology*. 3rd ed. Philadelphia, PA: Lippincott Williams & Wilkins. 1999;783:2516.
5. Conti JB, Belardinelli L, Curtis AB. Usefulness of adenosine in diagnosis of tachyarrhythmias. *Am J Cardiol*. 1995;75:952–955.
6. Chauhan VS, Krahn AD, Klein GJ, Skanes AC, Yee R. Supraventricular tachycardia. *Med Clin North Am*. 2001;85:193–223.
7. Woeber KA. Thyrotoxicosis and the heart. *N Engl J Med*. 1992;327:94–8.
8. Klein I, Ojamaa K. Thyrotoxicosis and the heart. *Endocrinol Metab Clin North Am*. 1998;27:51–62.
9. Rude RK, Oldham SB, Singer FR, Nicoloff JT. Treatment of thyrotoxic hypercalcemia with propranolol. *N Engl J Med*. 1976;294:431.
10. Burnam KD, Monchik JM, Earll JM, Wartofsky L. Ionized and total plasma calcium and parathyroid hormone in hyperthyroidism. *Ann Intern Med*. 1976;84:668.
11. Edelson GW, Kleerekoper M. Hypercalcemic crisis. *Med Clin North Am*. 1995;79:79–92.
12. Barsotti MM, Targovnik JH, Verso TA. Thyrotoxicosis, hypercalcemia, and secondary hyperparathyroidism. *Arch Intern Med*. 1979;139:661–663.
13. Rose BD, Post TW. *Clinical Physiology of Acid-Base and Electrolyte Disorders*. 5th ed. New York: McGraw-Hill; 2001:754–758.

CHAPTER 5

FISHING FOR A DIAGNOSIS

COLIN R. COOKE
Division of Pulmonary and Critical Care Medicine, University of Michigan, Ann Arbor, Michigan

JOHN V. L. SHEFFIELD
Division of General Medicine, Harborview Medical Center, University of Washington, Seattle, Washington

JAN V. HIRSCHMANN
Division of General Medicine, Veterans Affairs Puget Sound Health Care System, University of Washington, Seattle, Washington

A 54-year-old man with hypertension and type 2 diabetes mellitus entered the Chest Pain Evaluation Unit of a teaching hospital after 12 hours of intermittent thoracic discomfort. The pain began during dinner and was sharp, band-like, and located beneath the sternum and across the entire chest. He had dyspnea but no diaphoresis or nausea. A recumbent position relieved the pain after dinner, but it recurred during the night and again the following morning. He did not smoke and had no family history of coronary artery disease.

A useful approach in evaluating acute chest pain is to employ a hierarchical differential diagnosis that emphasizes life-threatening disorders requiring prompt recognition and intervention. Most prominent are cardiac ischemia, pericardial tamponade, pneumothorax, pulmonary embolus, esophageal rupture, and aortic dissection. The concurrent dyspnea and retrosternal location and the intermittent nature of the pain that this patient has are consistent with myocardial ischemia, but the sharp quality of the pain and the relief gained by being recumbent are atypical. Pain with pericarditis is characteristically pleuritic and often worse when lying down. The pain of pneumothorax is typically unilateral, not intermittent, and unlikely to improve with recumbency. Although pain during eating suggests the possibility of an esophageal source, spontaneous rupture usually follows vomiting. The pain is typically continuous and severe. The pain of pulmonary embolism may be unilateral and pleuritic but often is more diffuse. Relief by recumbency is unusual, but the intermittent nature could suggest recurrent emboli. The patient has a history of hypertension, which predisposes him to aortic dissection, in which the pain is typically sharp, continuous, and severe but occasionally intermittent. Among numerous less urgent diagnoses are esophagitis and thoracic diabetic radiculopathy.

Important features to look for during this patient's examination include disappearance of the radial pulse during inhalation, a simple screening test that is insensitive but very specific for pericardial tamponade; elevated neck veins, which can occur with tension pneumothorax, massive pulmonary embolism, and pericardial tamponade; pericardial and

Clinical Care Conundrums: Challenging Diagnoses in Hospital Medicine, First Edition.
Edited by James C. Pile, Thomas E. Baudendistel, and Brian J. Harte.

pleural friction rubs; discrepant blood pressures in both the arms, sometimes a sign of aortic dissection; local thoracic tenderness from chest wall disorders; and sensory examination of the chest surface, which is often abnormal in diabetic thoracic radiculopathy. Given the patient's age and history of diabetes, I am most concerned about myocardial ischemia. The most appropriate diagnostic tests include an electrocardiogram and a chest radiograph.

The patient appeared apprehensive but reported no pain. He had a temperature of 36.0°C, heart rate of 95 beats per minute, blood pressure of 138/77 mm Hg, respiratory rate of 16 breaths per minute, and oxygen saturation of 99% while breathing ambient air. Blood pressures were equal in both arms. Jugular venous distention was absent, and the lung and cardiac examinations were normal. His pain did not increase on chest wall palpation. Examination of the abdomen, extremities, and the neurologic system was normal.

Laboratory tests showed a leukocyte count of 12,700/mm^3, with 85% neutrophils, 8% lymphocytes, 6% monocytes, and 1% eosinophils. The hematocrit was 45%, and the platelet count was 172,000/mm^3. A basic chemistry panel was remarkable only for a glucose of 225 mg/dL. An electrocardiogram (ECG) showed a normal sinus rhythm and left anterior fascicular block without acute ST- or T-wave changes. Prior ECGs were unavailable. An anteroposterior radiograph disclosed low lung volumes and bibasilar opacities. No pleural effusion was noted. Serial serum troponin and creatine kinase levels were normal. A Tc 99m tetrofosmin cardiac nuclear perfusion test performed at rest demonstrated a moderate area of mildly decreased uptake along the inferior wall extending to the apex. An exercise treadmill test, terminated after 1 minute, 45 seconds because of chest pain, provoked no ECG changes diagnostic of ischemic disease.

The absence of elevated jugular venous pressure virtually eliminates pericardial tamponade as a diagnosis, and the chest film excludes pneumothorax. The intermittent nature of the chest pain; the absence on the chest radiograph of findings such as mediastinal gas, left pneumothorax, or hydropneumothorax; and the lack of a predisposing cause make esophageal rupture unlikely. Pulmonary embolism remains a consideration despite the normal oxygen saturation because hypoxemia is absent in a substantial minority of such cases. The normal cardiac enzyme levels and the lack of significant changes on the ECG exclude the possibility that a myocardial infarction has recently occurred, but cardiac ischemia remains a possibility, especially because the patient had chest pain on exercise and the nuclear scan indicated diminished blood flow to the inferior left ventricle. Aortic dissection still remains as a possibility. The inferior wall abnormalities seen on the scan could result from dissection into the right coronary artery, which is more frequently involved than the left, or compression of it by an enlarged aorta, but they may also be artifacts. The leukocytosis may be a nonspecific response to stress but could indicate, although unlikely, infections such as mediastinitis from esophageal rupture or bacterial aortitis.

A conscientious clinician would repeat the history, reexamine the patient, and scrutinize the chest film to determine what the bilateral opacities represent. Given the story so far, however, I might consider a thoracic computed tomography (CT) angiogram because I am most concerned about pulmonary emboli and aortic dissection.

On hospital day 3, the patient had worsening dyspnea and persistent chest pain. His temperature was 39.3°C, and his oxygen saturation decreased to 89% while breathing room air. Repeat chest radiography showed new bilateral pleural effusions and increased bibasilar opacification (Fig. 5.1). His leukocyte count

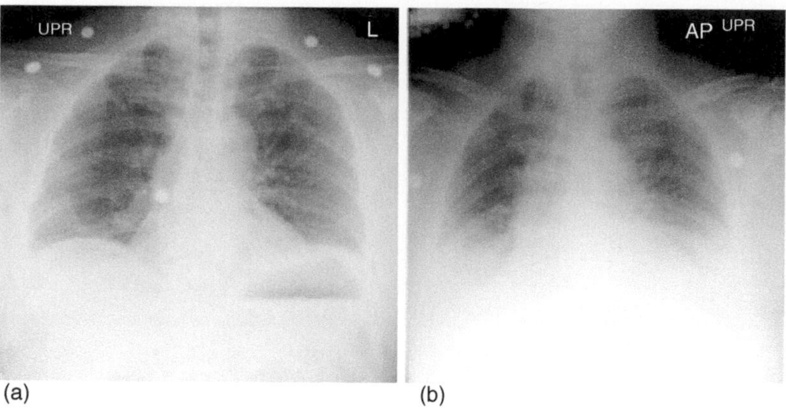

FIGURE 5.1 Anteroposterior chest radiographs on admission (a) and hospital day 3 (b) showing development of bibasilar opacities and bilateral pleural effusions.

was 19,000/mm^3, with 88% neutrophils, 6% lymphocytes, 5% monocytes, and 1% eosinophils. Care was transferred from the chest pain team to an inpatient general medicine team. A pulmonary CT angiogram showed no large central clots but suggested emboli in the right superior subsegmental artery and a right upper lobe subsegmental artery. Bilateral pleural effusions were observed, as were bilateral pleural-based atelectasis or infiltrates in the lower lungs. A hiatal hernia was noted, but no aortic dissection. The patient received supplemental oxygen, intravenous levofloxacin, and unfractionated heparin by continuous infusion.

I will assume that the fever is part of the patient's original disease and not a nosocomial infection or drug fever. At this point, a crucial part of the evaluation is examining the CT scan with experienced radiologists to determine whether the abnormalities noted are genuinely convincing for pulmonary emboli. If the findings are equivocal, the next step might be a pulmonary angiogram or the indirect approach of evaluating the leg veins with ultrasound, reasoning that the presence of proximal leg vein thromboses would require anticoagulation in any event.

The patient's worsening chest pain and hypoxemia are consistent with multiple pulmonary emboli. Bilateral pleural effusions and leukocytosis can occur with pulmonary embolism, but are uncommon. Because of the fever, another possibility is septic pulmonary emboli, but he has no evidence of suppurative thrombophlebitis of the peripheral veins, apparent infection elsewhere, or previous intravenous drug abuse causing right-sided endocarditis. An alternative diagnosis is infection of an initially bland pulmonary infarct.

Thoracentesis could provide additional diagnostic information depending on how persuasive the CT diagnosis of pulmonary embolism is and the size of the pleural effusions. It should be done before instituting antimicrobial therapy, which may decrease the yield of the cultures, and before starting heparin, which increases the risk of bleeding and occasionally causes a substantial, even fatal hemothorax.

The patient's oxygenation and dyspnea did not improve. Over the next day, he repeatedly mentioned that swallowing, particularly solid foods, worsened his chest pain. He had a temperature of 39.9°C, a heart rate of 121 beats per minute, blood pressure of 149/94 mm Hg, a respiratory rate of 28 per minute, and oxygen saturation of 93% while breathing 40% oxygen. He had inspiratory splinting, percussive dullness at both lung bases, and distant heart sounds. A contrast esophagogram

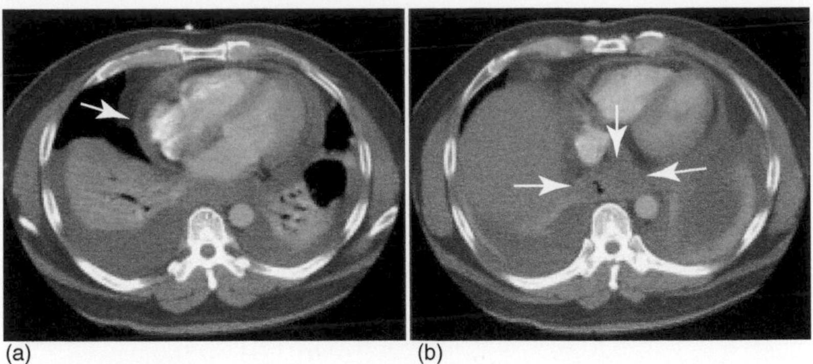

FIGURE 5.2 Repeat CT of chest showing pericardial effusion (a, arrow) and soft tissue esophageal mass (b, arrows).

showed distal narrowing that prevented solid contrast from passing, but no hiatal hernia. Blood and urine cultures obtained before antibiotic therapy were sterile. Duplex ultrasonography of bilateral lower extremities showed no evidence of deep venous thrombosis. A pulmonary angiogram revealed no emboli, and heparin was discontinued. Bilateral thoracentesis yielded grossly bloody fluid. Repeat chest CT (Fig. 5.2) demonstrated large bilateral effusions, a new large pericardial effusion, and a prominence at the gastroesophageal junction more concerning for a soft tissue mass than for a hiatal hernia, although the quality of the study was suboptimal because of the absence of oral contrast.

The CT scan now suggests a paraesophageal abscess from an esophageal rupture. As mentioned earlier, if rupture occurs spontaneously, it typically follows retching or vomiting and is called *Boerhaave's syndrome*. Another consideration is a rupture secondary to an external insult, such as trauma or ingestion of a caustic substance. In evaluating these possibilities, the patient should have been asked four questions at the initial interview that I neglected to explicitly highlight earlier. First, what was he eating when he developed the chest pain? Second, did the pain begin during swallowing? Third, did he have previous symptoms suggesting an esophageal disorder such as dysphagia, odynophagia, or heartburn? These might indicate a cancer that could perforate or another problem such as a stricture or disordered esophageal motility that might have caused a swallowed item to lodge in the esophagus. Finally, did he have retching or vomiting? Although not routinely part of the review of systems, the first two questions are an appropriate line of questioning of a patient with onset of chest pain while eating.

At this point, a reasonable approach would be an esophagoscopy to delineate any intraluminal problems, such as a cancer or a foreign body. The apparent obstruction seen on barium swallow may be from extrinsic pressure from a paraesophageal abscess. The patient should receive broad-spectrum antimicrobial therapy effective against oral anaerobes. Although occasionally patients recover with antibiotics alone, surgery is usually required. I am surprised that the original CT scan did not show evidence of an esophageal perforation. Possibly, the "hiatal hernia" was a paraesophageal abscess poorly characterized because of the lack of oral contrast.

The team, concerned about esophageal perforation, began the patient on intravenous clindamycin. The patient underwent video-assisted thoracoscopic drainage, which yielded a moderate amount of turbid, bloody fluid from each hemithorax. The pericardium contained approximately 500 cm^3 of turbid fluid. Gram stain and culture of these fluids were negative. No esophageal or mediastinal mass was noted during surgery. Intraoperative esophagogastroduodenoscopy with

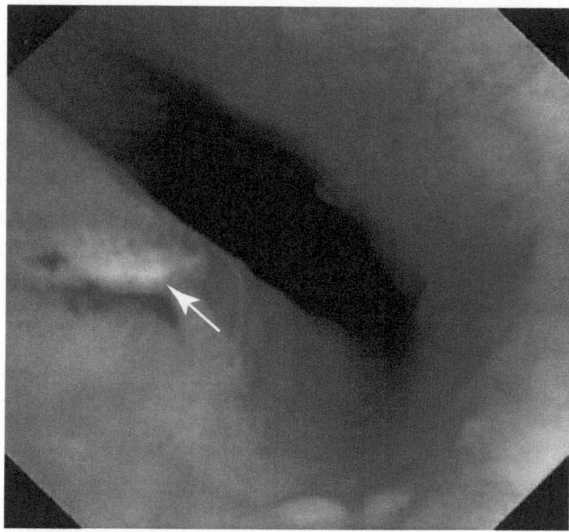

FIGURE 5.3 View of distal esophagus via endoscope showing a healing mucosal linear tear (arrow) at the site of the presumed esophageal perforation.

endoscopic ultrasound showed a healing linear mucosal tear in the distal esophagus (Fig. 5.3) as well as air/fluid collection in the esophageal soft tissue (not shown).

On further questioning postoperatively, the patient reported eating bony fish during the dinner when he first experienced chest pain. The patient received a 21-day course of oral clindamycin and completely recovered. Five weeks later, a chest CT showed decreased distal esophageal thickening and no mediastinal air.

COMMENTARY

Esophageal perforation is an uncommon but life-threatening cause of chest pain. In most series, iatrogenic injury accounts for more than 70% of cases, whereas most of the other cases have spontaneous (5%–20%) or traumatic (4%–10%) causes (Table 5.1).[1–4] Perforation as a complication of ingesting fish bones, although rare, is well described and continues to be reported.[5–7]

TABLE 5.1 Frequency of Causes of Esophageal Perforation

Etiology	Percentage (%)
Iatrogenic	45–77
Rigid or flexible endoscopy, balloon dilation, Blakemore tube, sclerotherapy, operative injury	
Increased intraesophageal pressure (Boerhaave's syndrome)	5–20
Vomiting or retching, weightlifting, childbirth	
Traumatic	4–10
Penetrating or blunt injury to neck or chest	
Ingestion	0–12
Foreign body, toxic or caustic substance	
Miscellaneous	0–5
Malignancy, Barrett's esophagus, infection, aortic dissection	

Data from references 1–4.

Diagnosis of esophageal perforation secondary to a foreign body may be difficult because of the considerable overlap of symptoms with other causes of chest pain and failure to consider this infrequent condition in the absence of a classic history of retching. Incorrectly evaluating or failing to obtain essential data can lead to incorrect or delayed diagnoses.

In the evaluation of this patient, the critical misstep was an incomplete history, both on arrival and when the patient was transferred to a second team. The presence of risk factors for coronary artery disease led the providers to first consider myocardial ischemia. They failed to ask crucial questions about the onset of the pain—when it occurred during the meal and what he was eating—even when the patient later complained of odynophagia. The providers, puzzled by the patient's ongoing and evolving symptoms, ordered numerous unnecessary diagnostic tests that gave false-positive results, leading to potentially harmful treatment including anticoagulation.

There is ongoing concern that the history-taking and physical examination skills of clinicians are in decline.[8–14] Many speculate this is in part due to reliance on increasingly sophisticated diagnostic tests, which providers may overly rely on because of their familiarity with the sensitivity and specificity of such tests, fear of malpractice litigation, diminishing opportunity to elucidate the complete history and physical exam, or lack of confidence in their history-taking and examination skills.[8–14] Although the rapid development and implementation of advanced diagnostic technologies have had a significant impact on diagnostic accuracy, the estimated rate of disease misdiagnosis remains as high as 24%.[15–18] In contrast to technology-based testing, the history and physical provide an inexpensive, safe, and effective means of arriving at a correct diagnosis. In outpatient medical visits, the history and physical, when completely elicited, result in a correct diagnosis of up to 70%–90% of patients.[8,19,20] Even for illnesses the diagnosis of which requires confirmation by a diagnostic test, the definitive test can only be selected after a sufficient history and exam provide an assessment of the pretest probability of disease.

In evaluating chest pain, there is an additional potential factor that diminishes reliance on bedside assessment. Modern quality assurance measures and chest pain units encourage clinicians to evaluate patients with chest pain quickly because any delay diminishes the benefits of therapies for acute coronary syndromes. In the emergency room, these patients find themselves on a rapidly moving diagnostic conveyor belt, an approach that is efficient and appropriate given the high prevalence of coronary disease but that also contributes to inattentiveness and error for patients with unusual diagnoses.

For most patients with chest pain, there is no finding that would change diagnostic probabilities enough to take them off the diagnostic conveyor belt. Nevertheless, several bedside findings can help providers to rank-order a differential diagnosis, thereby improving the sequence in which diagnostic testing is done. For patients with chest pain, the ECG has the highest predictive ability of all studied history, physical exam, and ECG findings (Table 5.2).[21] A history of "sharp" and "positional" pain descriptors diminishes the probability of myocardial ischemia.[21] Unfortunately, no history, exam, or ECG feature is sensitive enough, either alone or in combination, to effectively rule out myocardial ischemia.

The history and exam can also facilitate differentiation of noncoronary causes of life-threatening chest pain. The dismal performance of individual bedside findings for pulmonary embolism has led to the development of quantitative D-dimer assays and objective methods based on bedside evaluation, including the widely used Wells Score.[22] This score can be used to classify patients as having low, medium, and high risk of pulmonary embolism, facilitating management decisions after diagnostic imaging is obtained.[23] Fewer than half of all patients with thoracic aortic dissection have classic exam findings; however, when present, they can appropriately raise the probability of

TABLE 5.2 Positive Likelihood Ratios for History, Exam, and Bedside Findings in Life-Threatening Causes of Chest Pain

Finding	Positive LR*
Myocardial Ischemia	
ST-segment elevation or Q wave	22
S3 gallop, blood pressure < 100 mm Hg, or ST-segment depression	3.0
Sharp or positional pain	0.3
Pulmonary Embolism	
Low clinical probability	0.2
Medium clinical probability	1.8
High clinical probability	17.1
Aortic Dissection	
Tearing or ripping pain	10.8
Focal neurologic deficits	6.6-33
Ipsilateral versus contralateral pulse deficit	5.7
Cardiac Tamponade	
Pulsus paradoxus >12 mm Hg	5.9
Esophageal Perforation	
Dysphagia, odynophagia, retching, vomiting, or subcutaneous emphysema	Unknown

* Likelihood ratios (LRs), defined as sensitivity/1 − specificity.
From references 11, 22, 24, and 26.

dissection higher on the differential diagnosis.[24] Importantly, no history or exam finding argues against dissection.[24] Most patients with cardiac tamponade will have elevated jugular venous pressure (76%–100%); however, poor interobserver agreement about this finding may decrease its detection.[11,25,26] As the discussant notes, total paradox, defined as the palpable pulse disappearing with inspiration, is an insensitive test for tamponade, present in only 23% of patients with the disorder. In contrast, an inspiratory drop in systolic blood pressure of more than 12 mm Hg should prompt consideration for tamponade.[11,26] Commonly taught features of esophageal perforation, including chest pain, dysphagia, odynophagia, prior retching or vomiting, subcutaneous emphysema, dyspnea, and pleural effusions, vary in their reported sensitivity, but their specificity is virtually never reported.[27]

Like most patients with chest pain, our patient lacked all these symptoms and signs, arguing for myocardial ischemia, although he had a few signs that argued against it (sharp and positional chest pain). After the initial CXR and ECG, further testing with cardiac biomarkers was appropriate, but a fundamental error was made in not returning to the patient's bedside to repeat the interview and examination after the cardiac biomarkers were found to be normal. Had this been done, several clues would have pushed esophageal perforation to the top of the differential diagnosis. Subsequent testing would have led to the correct diagnosis and avoided a potentially harmful diagnostic "fishing expedition."

Key Points

1. Esophageal perforation is an uncommon but life-threatening cause of chest pain that is difficult to diagnose because of its nonspecific symptoms.
2. An accurate and complete history and exam can reveal signs and symptoms that influence the likelihood of each life-threatening cause of chest pain. Evaluating patients

for these features is vital to the rank-ordering of a differential diagnosis and the selection of appropriate diagnostic tests.

3. There is no substitute for repeating the history, reexamining the patient, and reevaluating available information when confronted with a confusing constellation of symptoms.

REFERENCES

1. Goldstein LA, Thompson WR. Esophageal perforations: a 15 year experience. *Am J Surg*. 1982;143: 495–503.
2. Bufkin BL, Miller JI Jr., Mansour KA. Esophageal perforation: emphasis on management. *Ann Thorac Surg*. 1996;61:1447–1451; discussion 1451–1452.
3. Brinster CJ, Singhal S, Lee L, Marshall MB, Kaiser LR, Kucharczuk JC. Evolving options in the management of esophageal perforation. *Ann Thorac Surg*. 2004;77:1475–1783.
4. Gupta NM, Kaman L. Personal management of 57 consecutive patients with esophageal perforation. *Am J Surg*. 2004;187:58–63.
5. D'Costa H, Bailey F, McGavigan B, George G, Todd B. Perforation of the oesophagus and aorta after eating fish: an unusual cause of chest pain. *Emerg Med J*. 2003;20:385–386.
6. Katsetos MC, Tagbo AC, Lindberg MP, Rosson RS. Esophageal perforation and mediastinitis from fish bone ingestion. *South Med J*. 2003;96:516–520.
7. Medina HM, Garcia MJ, Velazquez O, Sandoval N. A 73-year-old man with chest pain 4 days after a fish dinner. *Chest*. 2004;126:294–297.
8. Sackett DL, Rennie D. The science of the art of the clinical examination. *JAMA*. 1992;267:2650–2652.
9. Li JT. Clinical skills in the 21st century. *Arch Intern Med*. 1994;154:22–24.
10. Mangione S, Nieman LZ. Pulmonary auscultatory skills during training in internal medicine and family practice. *Am J Respir Crit Care Med*. 1999;159:1119–1124.
11. McGee SR. *Evidence-based physical diagnosis*. Philadelphia, PA: Saunders; 2001.
12. Schattner A. Simple is beautiful: the neglected power of simple tests. *Arch Intern Med*. 2004;164: 2198–2200.
13. Schattner A, Fletcher RH. Pearls and pitfalls in patient care: need to revive traditional clinical values. *Am J Med Sci*. 2004;327:79–85.
14. Thompson GR III, Verghese A. Physical diagnosis: a lost art? Agency for Health Research and Quality. *WebM&M (Morbidity and Mortality Rounds on the Web)*. Medicine, August 2006. Available at: http://www.webmm.ahrq.gov/case.aspx?caseID=131. Accessed November 30, 2012.
15. Kirch W, Schafii C. Misdiagnosis at a university hospital in 4 medical eras. *Medicine (Baltimore)*. 1996;75:29–40.
16. Lundberg GD. Low-tech autopsies in the era of high-tech medicine: continued value for quality assurance and patient safety. *JAMA*. 1998;280:1273–1274.
17. Flum DR, Morris A, Koepsell T, Dellinger EP. Has misdiagnosis of appendicitis decreased over time? A population-based analysis. *JAMA*. 2001;286:1748–1753.
18. Shojania KG, Burton EC, McDonald KM, Goldman L. Changes in rates of autopsy-detected diagnostic errors over time: a systematic review. *JAMA*. 2003;289:2849–2856.
19. Crombie DL. Diagnostic process. *J Coll Gen Pract*. 1963;54:579–589.
20. Sandler G. The importance of the history in the medical clinic and the cost of unnecessary tests. *Am Heart J*. 1980;100:928–931.
21. Chun AA, McGee SR. Bedside diagnosis of coronary artery disease: a systematic review. *Am J Med*. 2004;117:334–343.
22. Wells PS, Ginsberg JS, Anderson DR, et al. Use of a clinical model for safe management of patients with suspected pulmonary embolism. *Ann Intern Med*. 1998;129:997–1005.
23. Stein PD, Woodard PK, Weg JG, et al. Diagnostic pathways in acute pulmonary embolism: recommendations of the PIO-PED II investigators. *Am J Med*. 2006;119:1048–1055.
24. Klompas M. Does this patient have an acute thoracic aortic dissection? *JAMA*. 2002;287:2262–2272.
25. Cook DJ, Simel DL. The rational clinical examination. Does this patient have abnormal central venous pressure? *JAMA*. 1996;275:630–634.
26. Roy CL, Minor MA, Brookhart MA, Choudhry NK. Does this patient with a pericardial effusion have cardiac tamponade? *JAMA*. 2007;297:1810–1818.
27. Lemke T, Jagminas L. Spontaneous esophageal rupture: a frequently missed diagnosis. *Am Surg*. 1999;65: 449–452.

CHAPTER **6**

A RASH DECISION

BRIAN J. HARTE

South Pointe Hospital, Cleveland Clinic Health System, Warrensville Heights, Ohio

GURPREET DHALIWAL

Department of Medicine, University of California, San Francisco, California; Medical Service, San Francisco VA Medical Center, San Francisco, California

WENDY ARMSTRONG

Department of Infectious Disease, Emory University School of Medicine, Atlanta, Georgia

JAMES C. PILE

Departments of Hospital Medicine and Infectious Diseases, Cleveland Clinic, Cleveland, Ohio

A 38-year-old HIV+ Ohio man with a recent CD4+ count of 534 cells/mL presented to his physician with 3 weeks of fever as high as 102°F. He noted mild myalgias, pruritus, and an occasional cough but no headache, sore throat, dyspnea, rash, or gastrointestinal or genitourinary complaints. He had been seen elsewhere 2 weeks previously, when he had reported a single episode of receptive oral sex with a male partner several weeks earlier. He had been prescribed ciprofloxacin and azithromycin, but a throat swab came back negative for *Chlamydia* and *Neisseria gonorrhoeae*, and he reported no change in his symptoms after the course of antibiotics. He denied smoking or using street drugs. His only medications were citalopram and trazodone for depression.

This is a HIV+ man with a mild degree of immunosuppression with a fever of unknown origin (FUO). It is not yet known if the requisite basic infectious evaluation has been completed to meet this definition, but the duration certainly qualifies, and regardless of semantics, the FUO framework is a helpful starting point. The primary considerations in FUO are infections, neoplasms, and autoimmune illnesses. Autoimmune diseases are relatively less common in HIV patients. Although pruritus is quite common in HIV alone, it may also herald renal failure, cholestasis, or a malignancy (usually hematologic). Drugs must also be considered as a cause of unexplained fever; the pruritus might suggest an allergic reaction, although citalopram or trazodone do not commonly have this effect. The failure to respond to broad-spectrum antimicrobials (along with the duration of illness) lowers my suspicion for common infections such as pneumonia, urinary tract infection, or cellulitis. Among sexually transmitted diseases, syphilis can be protean and merits consideration.

Clinical Care Conundrums: Challenging Diagnoses in Hospital Medicine, First Edition.
Edited by James C. Pile, Thomas E. Baudendistel, and Brian J. Harte.

On examination, he appeared well. His temperature was 102.4°F; pulse, 111 beats per minute; and blood pressure, 138/78 mm Hg. The head, neck, cardiovascular system, and lungs appeared normal on examination. The abdomen was soft and nontender without organomegaly; skin, extremities, and neurological system were unremarkable. Rectal examination showed small anal condylomata. Hemoglobin was 14.3 g/dL; white blood cell count, 6200/cm^3; and platelet count, 230,000/cm^3. Serum electrolytes and lactate dehydrogenase were normal. The results of his liver function tests (LFTs) **demonstrated the following: serum aspartate transaminase, 60 U/L (normal, 7–40 U/L); alanine transaminase, 125 U/L (normal, 5–50 U/L); alkaline phosphatase, 218 U/L (normal, 40–150 U/L); and total bilirubin, 2.1 mg/dL (normal, 0.0–1.5 mg/dL). Urinalysis demonstrated 2+ bilirubin and was otherwise normal. His erythrocyte sedimentation rate was 32 mm/hour (normal, 0–15 mm/hour).**

After 3 weeks of illness, his CBC demonstrated no signs of chronic illness (such as anemia of a chronic disease or a reactive leukocytosis or thrombocytosis). The results of his LFTs showed moderate elevation, slightly more cholestatic than hepatocellular. This finding may reflect a disease process involving the liver, but such abnormal findings are often nonspecific in acute and chronic illnesses. With an unremitting fever, infectious complications in the liver merit early consideration. The time course rules out common biliary disorders such as cholangitis or cholecystitis. Pyogenic or amoebic liver abscesses are possible (homosexual men are at increased risk for the latter), but the absence of pain or abdominal tenderness is atypical. This biochemical profile can also be seen in chronic (but not acute) viral infections of the liver. Chronic hepatitis B and C predispose to hepatocellular carcinoma (HCC), which can be associated with fever. Cancers that infiltrate the liver, such as lymphoma or carcinoma, could also account for this picture. Indolent infections such as tuberculosis (TB) and syphilis are also possible, so associated signs of these systemic diseases should be sought. I do not believe either of his antibiotics is commonly associated with LFT abnormalities, and his CD4 count is too high for HIV cholangiopathy. In sum, a host of liver diseases are possible, but an extrahepatic systemic disease deserves equal attention.

His CD4+ count was 537 cells/mL, and his HIV RNA viral load was 44,300 copies/mL. Radiographs of the chest were normal. Two sets of blood cultures were negative. The rapid plasma reagin (RPR) **was nonreactive. The results of serologies for acute hepatitis A, B, C, and E; chronic hepatitis B and C; and toxoplasmosis were negative. Testing for both Epstein–Barr virus and cytomegalovirus showed evidence of remote infection. Results of serologies for *Bartonella* species, human herpesviruses 6 and 7, and parvovirus B19 were negative.**

The negative RPR makes disseminated (secondary) syphilis improbable, provided the prozone phenomenon has been excluded. An extensive serological workup is common in the evaluation of FUO, although the threat of false-positive results always looms when many studies are sent simultaneously. This must be considered in advance here, as his relatively preserved CD4 count affords him significant protection against many opportunistic infections. His HIV infection, however, regardless of CD4 count, increases his risk for TB and lymphoma, which remain high on my list. Both may be residing primarily in the liver. In FUO, the abdominal CT is frequently a high-yield test (primarily by demonstrating unsuspected tumors and abscesses), even in the absence of symptoms, and would certainly be of interest here given the LFT results. Imaging could diagnose febrile tumors such as lymphoma, HCC, or renal cell carcinoma. In the event that imaging is unrevealing, causes of granulomatous hepatitis should be entertained. The constellation

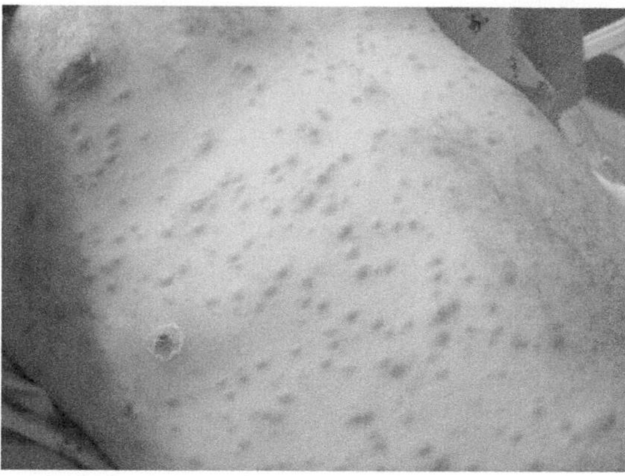

FIGURE 6.1 Truncal rash.

of cough, LFT abnormalities, and fever is compatible with Q fever. As with any FUO case, I would also carefully revisit this patient's history to discern where he was born, where he has been, and what activities or exposures he is engaged in.

He was seen 2 days later with fever of 104°F and new papules over his sternal area. Over the next week, he had intermittent fevers and severe fatigue. The rash progressed, predominantly involving his chest and back, but also his legs, arms, and face (Fig. 6.1). The lesions spared his palms and soles. The exanthem was intensely pruritic and maculopapular, consisting of lesions with a diameter of 0.5 cm or less, with some scaling. There were no vesicles or pustular lesions. There were no other new findings on examination. His transaminase and bilirubin had normalized, and his CBC and electrolytes were unchanged. Repeat blood cultures held for extended incubation were negative. Computerized tomography of the chest, abdomen, and pelvis demonstrated mild lymphadenopathy at the porta hepatis with increased portocaval and periaortic lymphadenopathy.

The only LFT abnormality that persists is the elevated alkaline phosphatase, which suggests that (i) liver involvement was not specific and that there is a disease process involving the bone; (ii) there is a persistent infiltrative disorder of the liver such as infection or malignancy or, less likely, amyloidosis or sarcoidosis; or (iii) the porta hepatis lymphadenopathy is causing biliary obstruction. The underlying diagnosis must explain the rash, intra-abdominal lymphadenopathy, and fever. The time course does somewhat limit the extensive differential of fever and rash. After 3 weeks of illness, some of the most life-threatening entities such as meningococcal disease, Rocky Mountain spotted fever, and toxic shock syndrome are unlikely. Concern remains for infections that are more indolent, such as mycobacteria, fungi, or spirochetes. The most striking elements of the rash are the extensive distribution, rapid progression, large number, and discreteness of the lesions, which collectively point more toward disseminated fungal (e.g., histoplasmosis, as he lives in Ohio), spirochetal, rickettsial, or viral etiologies, rather than bacterial or mycobacterial entities. The absence of vesicles detracts from the diagnosis of a disseminated herpesvirus such as herpes simplex or varicella. I believe that this rash is too disseminated to be caused by a common mycobacterial illness. This extent of cutaneous metastases would usually accompany a far more ill patient with an obvious primary cancer (none is seen on imaging in this patient), and it appears too extensive to be caused by a paraneoplastic phenomenon such as Sweet's syndrome. A systemic vasculitis or another autoimmune disease remains possible, but there is minimal evidence of visceral organ involvement. All the aforementioned diseases could explain the intra-abdominal lymphadenopathy, but my suspicion is highest for infection. I would biopsy and culture the skin lesions, repeat the RPR and/or send a treponemal-specific test, place a PPD skin test, and send fungal studies (serum serologies and urine antigens) for evaluation. If the results of these noninvasive studies are unrevealing, I would consider a liver biopsy.

The patient's medications were discontinued, and a skin biopsy of the rash from his chest showed atypical lymphohistiocytic infiltrates without acute inflammatory cells and with negative Gomori methenamine silver (GMS), **acid-fast bacilli** (AFB), **and the Fite (for *Nocardia*) stains. The infiltrates were predominantly T cells with a 1:1 CD4/CD8 ratio. This was read as suspicious for cytotoxic (CD8) mycosis fungoides.**

I do not have reason to doubt the pathologist's impression of mycosis fungoides on histopathologic grounds, but from a clinical standpoint, I do not think mycosis fungoides is a disease that has a prolonged febrile prodrome or an explosive cutaneous onset. Rather, it is frequently preceded by nonspecific skin findings over a long period. Thinking broadly and pathophysiologically and noting that T cells are the predominant lymphocytes in skin, I wonder if they could represent a nonmalignant, immunological reaction in the skin. The stains, although not perfectly sensitive, make mycobacterial and fungal diseases less likely; however, incubation of cultures is necessary.

Over the next 10 days (bringing the total duration of the patient's illness to 6 weeks), the skin lesions increased in number. In the physician's office at his next follow-up, the patient had a temperature of 104.1°F, was uncomfortable, shivering, and ill-appearing. His blood pressure was 108/66 mm Hg, and his pulse was 114 beats per minute. He complained of severe shooting pains, predominantly in his pretibial regions and arms. Examination showed no other new findings, including no focal neurological findings. The results of the T-cell rearrangement study from the skin biopsy showed evidence of a monoclonal T-cell population. He was admitted to the hospital for further evaluation and treatment.

The extremity dysesthesias could represent a lesion of the spinal cord (including the CSF/meninges), a polyradiculopathy, or a polyneuropathy. Unfortunately, this does not add a tremendous amount of diagnostic resolution, as infection, malignancy, and autoimmune syndromes, such as vasculitis, may all involve the nervous system in these ways. In general, I associate monoclonal lymphocyte responses with hematological malignancies and polyclonal responses with the less specific inflammation that could accompany infection, autoimmunity, or solid malignancies. His age, fever, and rapid progression seem atypical for mycosis fungoides, but given the monoclonal T cells, this must now be considered. Adult T-cell leukemia/lymphoma, with its prominent skin manifestations and its association with HLTV-1, is an alternative T-cell malignancy that could explain the fever, neurological symptoms, and possible visceral involvement (elevated alkaline phosphatase, which could reflect liver or bone). In cases that are diagnostic challenges, one of the highest-yield maneuvers is to repeat the preceding evaluation, starting with the history, exam, and basic labs, and if necessary, to review or repeat the imaging or skin biopsy. Given the elevated alkaline phosphatase, disseminated rash, new neurological symptoms, and his HIV status, I remain particularly concerned about syphilis and would do further testing (accounting for the prozone phenomenon) before proceeding with the malignancy evaluation.

A lumbar puncture demonstrated clear cerebrospinal fluid, with 2 leukocytes and 195 erythrocytes/cm^3, protein of 26 mg/dL, and glucose of 52 mg/dL. Bacterial

and fungal cultures of the fluid were negative. The results of colonoscopy were normal. A bone marrow biopsy demonstrated ring granulomas. GMS, AFB, Fite, and Steiner (for spirochetes) stains were negative, cultures of the aspirate were negative for bacteria, and smears were negative for fungi and mycobacteria. Antibody tests for human T-cell lymphotropic virus types I and II, *Coxiella burnetii*, and *Bartonella henselae* were negative. The dermatology consultant believed the absence of lymphadenopathy and the pruritic nature of the lesions were atypical for cytotoxic T-cell lymphoma (CTCL). Before initiating therapy for CTCL, the dermatology consultant suggested repeating the skin biopsy and RPR.

The repeat RPR was positive at 1:64 dilutions, and a confirmatory fluorescent treponemal antibody absorption test showed a positive result. He was prescribed intramuscular benzathine pencillin 2.4 million units weekly for 3 weeks, with almost immediate defervescence and slower resolution of his rash and shooting pains in his limbs.

The repeat skin biopsy done during the hospitalization demonstrated lichenoid-type dermatitis with interstitial and perivascular lymphohistiocytic infiltrates and granulomas. Steiner stains for spirochetes were positive. Immunohistochemical stains ruled out a lymphoproliferative process. One year later, his RPR was nonreactive.

COMMENTARY

FUO was first defined by Petersdorf and Beeson in 1961 as a temperature higher than 38.3°C on several occasions lasting longer than 3 weeks and defying diagnosis despite 1 week of inpatient investigation.[1] Dramatic changes in medical practice have rendered this definition outdated, with more recent proposals allowing thoughtful outpatient investigation to serve as a surrogate for hospitalization. Some have proposed that HIV-associated FUO be considered a distinct entity, with the most complete North American series finding the etiology of the HIV-associated FUO in 56 of 70 patients.[2] The mean CD4+ count in this series was 58/mm^3. Disseminated *Mycobacterium avium* was the most frequently diagnosed cause, followed by *Pneumocystis jirovecii* pneumonia, cytomegalovirus infection, disseminated histoplasmosis, and lymphoma. Of 14 patients with fever of no definable etiology, 12 eventually proved to have self-limiting illness.

Despite numerous attempts to reduce the investigation of the patient with FUO to an algorithm, the approach must be individualized. A thorough history and careful serial physical examinations are frequently and appropriately stressed as the foundation, followed by thoughtful selection of laboratory and imaging studies. Although FUO has a lengthy differential diagnosis, it often proves to be an unusual manifestation of a common disease, rather than a typical presentation of a rare disease.[3] A relatively uncommon disease in conjunction with an initially negative diagnostic test result, as was the case with this patient, may lead to a protracted diagnostic puzzle.

Syphilis is a rare cause of FUO. In six large studies of a total of 947 patients published over a 40-year period, only two cases of syphilis (one secondary and one neurosyphilis) were reported.[1,4–8] Syphilis as a cause of prolonged cryptic fever appears to have been seen with greater frequency in the preantibiotic era.[9] In the first half of the 20th century, syphilis was known as the great imitator, with its unusual manifestations recognized and indeed expected. As a result of the dramatically lower incidence of syphilis in recent decades, these lessons have largely been forgotten, which may lead to diagnostic confusion when syphilis presents atypically. The manifestations of secondary syphilis are protean, including a variety of rashes, aphthous ulcers, arthralgias, pharyngitis, weight loss, fever, meningitis, ocular symptoms, cranial nerve palsies, glomerulonephritis, hepatitis, and periostitis (which afflicted this patient, who complained of "severe shooting pains" in his arms and shins).

After declining in the last decade of the 20th century, the rates of primary and secondary syphilis are rising in the United States.[10] Oral sex is a clear risk factor for syphilis transmission, particularly for men who have sex with men.[11] Because of the patient's exposure history and clinical picture, his outpatient physician considered the diagnosis of secondary syphilis early in the course of his illness. The diagnosis was not entertained further when the RPR test, highly sensitive at this stage of the disease, returned nonreactive. Likewise, when a rash subsequently appeared, the lack of palm and sole involvement dissuaded multiple clinicians from reconsidering the diagnosis of syphilis. A skin biopsy that appeared to lead in a distinctly different direction understandably confused the picture still further. Even at the time of the lumbar puncture, VDRL of the CSF was not ordered.

In retrospect, the chief confounder in the case was the false-negative RPR test, as the discussant suspected early on. Although nontreponemal tests are generally accurate in individuals with HIV, delayed seropositivity and false-negatives have been reported in this population.[12] The false-negative could have also been a result of the prozone phenomenon, an unusual event, occurring in fewer than 2% of cases of secondary syphilis and attributed to a mismatch between antibody and very high antigen level. The prozone reaction can be corrected for by requesting dilution of the serum prior to repeating the test. Simple lab error must be considered as well, but without access to this patient's serum from his original testing, the cause of his initial false-negative test cannot be known with certainty.

An unusual presentation in conjunction with failure to recognize the causes of rare false-negative testing for secondary syphilis led to a delayed diagnosis in this patient. Although syphilis and mycosis fungoides have previously been reported to mimic one another both clinically and histopathologically, the potential for secondary syphilis to be misdiagnosed in this fashion is not generally appreciated.[13–15] Recognition of the possibility of secondary syphilis occurred just in time to spare this patient the "rash decision" of treating him with cytotoxic therapy directed against CTCL.

Key Points

1. HIV-associated FUO can be a diagnostic challenge, but an etiology can be found in most cases.
2. Syphilis continues to be an unusual cause of FUO and can have protean manifestations affecting nearly every organ system.
3. The sensitivity of RPR is extremely high in secondary syphilis, but false-negative tests can be seen in HIV because of both the prozone phenomenon and a delayed rise in antibodies.

REFERENCES

1. Petersdorf RG, Beeson PB. Fever of unexplained origin: Report on 100 cases. *Medicine*. 1961;40:1–30.
2. Armstrong WS, Katz KT, Kazanjian PH. Human immunodeficiency virus-associated fever of unknown origin: A study of 70 patients in the United States and review. *Clin Infect Dis*. 1999;28:341–345.
3. Mackowiak PA, Durack DT. Fever of unknown origin. In: Mandell GL, Bennett JE, Dolin R, eds. *Principles and Practice of Infectious Diseases*. 6th ed. Philadelphia: Elsevier Churchill Livingstone; 2005:718–729.

4. Larson EB, Featherstone HJ, Petersdorf RG. Fever of unknown origin: Diagnosis and follow-up of 105 cases, 1970-1980. *Medicine*. 1982;61:269–292.
5. Knockaert DC, Vanneste LJ, Vanneste SB, Bobbaers JH. Fever of unknown origin in the 1980s: An update of the diagnostic spectrum. *Arch Intern Med*. 1992;152:51–55.
6. Kazanjian, PH. Fever of unknown origin: Review of 86 patients treated in community hospitals. *Clin Infect Dis*. 1992;15:968–973.
7. de Kleijn EM, van Lier HJ, van der Meer JW. Fever of unknown origin (FUO). I. A prospective multicenter study of 167 patients with FUO, using fixed epidemiologic entry criteria. The Netherlands FUO study group. *Medicine*. 1997;76:392–400.
8. Vanderschueren S, Knockaert D, Adriaenssens T, et al. From prolonged febrile illness to fever of unknown origin: The challenge continues. *Arch Intern Med*. 2003;163:1033–1041.
9. Hamman L, Wainright CW. The diagnosis of obscure fever. II. The diagnosis of unexplained high fever. *Bull Johns Hopkins Hosp*. 1936;58:307–331.
10. Centers for Disease Control and Prevention. Primary and secondary syphilis—United States, 2003–2004. *MMWR Morb Mortal Wkly Rep*. 2006;55:269–273.
11. Centers for Disease Control and Prevention. Transmission of primary and secondary syphilis by oral sex—Chicago, Illinois, 1998-2202. *MMWR Morb Mortal Wkly Rep*. 2004;53:966–968.
12. Kingston AA, Vujevich J, Shapiro M, et al. Seronegative secondary syphilis in 2 patients coinfected with human immunodeficiency virus. *Arch Dermatol*. 2005;141:431–433.
13. Levin DL, Greenberg MH, Hasegawa J, Roenigk HH. Secondary syphilis mimicking mycosis fungoides. *J Am Acad Dermatol*. 1980;3:92–94.
14. D'Amico R, Zalusky R. A case of lues maligna in a patient with acquired immunodeficiency syndrome (AIDS). *Scand J Infect Dis*. 2005;37:697–700.
15. Liotta EA, Turiansky GW, Berberian BJ, Sulica VI, Tomaszewski MM. Unusual presentation of secondary syphilis in 2 HIV-1 positive patients. *Cutis*. 2000;66:383–389.

CHAPTER 7

ONE HUNDRED YEARS LATER

THOMAS E. BAUDENDISTEL

Department of Medicine, Kaiser Permanente Medical Center, Oakland, California

NIMA AFSHAR and LAWRENCE M. TIERNEY JR.

Department of Medicine, University of California, San Francisco, California

A 36-year-old male physician was admitted to a Baltimore hospital in April 1907 with weight loss, weakness, arthralgias, and abdominal distension that had progressed over 5 years.

In 1907, major causes of unexplained weight loss included tuberculosis, hyperthyroidism, cancer, and diabetes. Arthralgias and weakness are not specific. The insidious progression over 5 years narrows the infectious possibilities; tuberculosis and syphilis are important considerations. Since surgical removal was the main treatment for malignancy in 1907, a history of prior surgery might point to a previously diagnosed malignancy that is now progressing.

Five years earlier, while visiting Turkey as a medical missionary, he first noted the onset of arthralgias that lasted 6–8 hours and occurred three to four times per week. Over time, these attacks lasted up to 24 hours and became associated with warmth, swelling, and tenderness of both small and large joints. He gradually lost weight and strength. One year prior to arrival in the hospital, he developed a cough productive of yellow sputum. Seven months prior, he returned from Turkey to Atlanta and noticed an increase in his cough, along with fevers of 100°F and night sweats.

The primacy of the arthralgias in this illness led me to consider primary rheumatic diseases and multisystem diseases (including infections) with a predominant skeletal component. In 1907, tests for lupus and the rheumatoid factor were not available. Neither skeletal remains nor works of art provide evidence that rheumatoid arthritis existed until the 19th century, whereas ankylosing spondylitis, gout, and rickets were present earlier.

As a medical missionary, he might have acquired a disease endemic to the areas he visited, or the travel history may be a red herring. Familial Mediterranean fever, although prevalent in Turkey and a cause of arthralgias accompanied by recurrent attacks of abdominal pain and fever, is not an acquired disease. Behcet's disease, also known as *Silk Trader's Route disease*, is found in ethnic populations of the countries that comprised the ancient Silk Route from Japan to the Middle East and may cause arthritis along with oral ulcers, genital lesions, pathergy, or uveitis. I would inquire about his ancestry and fevers before dismissing these possibilities.

Clinical Care Conundrums: Challenging Diagnoses in Hospital Medicine, First Edition.
Edited by James C. Pile, Thomas E. Baudendistel, and Brian J. Harte.

Although 5 years would be unusually long for tuberculosis to go unrecognized, a physician in the first half of the 20th century would place tuberculosis near the top of possible diagnoses. In 1930, a time when the population of the United States was considerably less, there were over 300,000 cases of tuberculosis. Physicians, and in particular pathologists since autopsies were more commonly performed, often died from tuberculosis because streptomycin, the first antituberculous medication, did not arrive until 1944. At the turn of the 20th century, the ability to detect tubercle bacilli was quite good. Thus, I would include tuberculous peritonitis as a cause of the progressive abdominal symptoms in this physician. In approximately one-third of patients with tuberculous peritonitis, there is evidence of pulmonary disease, and I would try to culture tubercle bacilli in the samples of sputum, a test then so common it probably rivaled our frequent complete blood counts in popularity.

Six months prior, examinations of sputum were negative for tubercle bacilli. Four months prior to arrival, the patient moved to New Mexico. His cough improved but he continued to lose weight and had diarrhea consisting of three to four loose or semiformed bowel movements per day. Three months prior to admission, he noted an increase in abdominal girth along with right lower quadrant fullness. One month prior, he noted painful swelling and warmth in both ankles, as well as dyspnea with exertion.

The increased abdominal girth in the context of chronic illness might be due to ascites, adenopathy, visceromegaly, or mass lesions such as a neoplasm or abscess. If ascites is the cause, one would need to consider primary hepatic disorders, as well as extrahepatic diseases that could progress over years. Infection with hepatitis A virus does not cause chronic liver disease. Hepatitis B, in those days, was referred to as *serum hepatitis*, and a serum marker for the B virus—the Australia antigen—was not identified until 1967. Cardiac causes of ascites include congestive heart failure and constrictive pericarditis, the latter an important consideration because it is potentially curable. Also, constrictive pericarditis can present as an indolent weight-losing disease because of chronic visceral congestion. Other considerations include nephrotic syndrome, infection, and neoplasm, including mesothelioma.

Abdominal distention might also be seen with a smoldering abscess. In addition to an appendiceal process, the travel and right lower quadrant localization reminds us to consider ameboma. This patient surely was in an area where amebiasis was endemic, and ameboma—a chronic inflammatory infection that is caused by *Entamoeba histolytica* and not associated with diarrhea or liver cysts—may mimic cecal carcinoma. Exertional dyspnea suggests at least the possibility of cardiac disease. Despite the negative sputum cultures, tuberculosis remains high on the list as a cause of constrictive pericarditis or peritonitis, either of which may occur in the absence of active pulmonary disease.

Past medical history included measles and whooping cough as a child, mild pleurisy at age 14, and mild influenza 7 years previously. The patient had a tonsillectomy as a child and had a portion of his inferior turbinate bone removed in an attempt to relieve a nasal condition.

On physical exam, the patient was thin and the skin over his face and hands was deep brown. His temperature was 101.5°F; heart rate, 100; and respiratory rate, 24. Small lymph nodes were palpable in the axillary and epitrochlear areas. His thorax moved asymmetrically, with less movement on the left apex and slight dullness to percussion in that area. The pulmonic component of the second heart sound was mildly accentuated. The abdomen displayed fullness and tympany, most pronounced in the right lower quadrant without hepatosplenomegaly. The left ankle

was swollen, and the overlying skin was tense, shiny, and hot. On both lower legs, areas of discoloration and slight induration were observed, felt to be consistent with faded erythema nodosum.

Although pleurisy has numerous causes, its presence raises the specter of tuberculosis again. The nasal condition triggers thoughts of Wegener's granulomatosis or lethal midline granuloma, both unlikely diagnoses here. The pulmonary exam suggests an apical process, such as tuberculosis, and the accentuated pulmonic heart sound implies pulmonary hypertension, which could be due to a number of chronic pulmonary diseases. The epitrochlear nodes are of interest since lymphoma and Hodgkin's disease rarely involve this area; syphilis and human immunodeficiency virus (HIV) infection are a few of the chronic diseases that may involve this lymph node region. More helpful is the absence of hepatosplenomegaly, since many indolent malignancies and infections would be expected to enlarge these organs by this point.

Monoarticular arthritis is often due to infection, and less likely due to rheumatoid disease. When rheumatoid arthritis flares, the entire skeleton flares, not single joints. Given the indolence and this single-joint involvement, tuberculosis again comes to mind.

I would next want to obtain a plain chest radiograph, looking for evidence of tuberculosis. As with any test, one should ask how this will change management. In 1907, antituberculous medications were not available, so therapy was directed at lowering oxygen tension in the primary site of infection; for example, pulmonary disease was addressed via pneumothorax. If the chest radiograph provides little hint of tuberculosis, then consideration must be given to exploratory surgery of the abdomen, given the focal abnormality in the right lower quadrant.

A peripheral blood smear revealed a hypochromic microcytic anemia. The total red blood cell count was 4.468 million/mm^3 (normal range for men is 4.52–5.90 million/mm^3) and white blood cell count was 8180/mm^3, including 80% granulocytes and 9% eosinophils. On gross inspection, the stool was clay-colored, and stool microscopy demonstrated large numbers of neutral fat droplets, but no ova, parasites, or tubercle bacilli. Urinalysis revealed no albumin or casts, and the bones were normal on ankle radiographs. Another sample of sputum revealed no tubercle bacilli, and intradermal placement of tuberculin provoked no reaction.

His negative tuberculin skin reaction is unusual for that era, because of the prevalence of tuberculosis. Most likely, he is anergic because of his severe underlying illness, and the absent reaction is thus not all that helpful a clue. Multiple negative sputum examinations lower the possibility of pulmonary, but not extrapulmonary, tuberculosis. The absence of bony destruction on ankle radiographs lowers my suspicion for tuberculous arthritis.

The excess stool fat implies steatogenic diarrhea from malabsorption, and two categories here are pancreatic and luminal diseases. Of these two categories, pancreatic etiologies produce more severe malabsorption. We do not hear mention of jaundice, however, and I cannot see how to link the pancreas to the arthritis. A chronic infection that may produce malabsorption and eosinophilia is strongyloidiasis, endemic in the southeastern United States. However, this patient did not manifest the most common finding of chronic strongyloidiasis, namely, asthma. Adrenal insufficiency, as might result from disseminated tuberculosis, is associated with increased skin pigmentation, diarrhea, and eosinophilia. However, the diarrhea of adrenal insufficiency is not malabsorptive, and serum electrolytes and cortisol tests were not available then to confirm this diagnosis antemortem.

In an attempt to identify a unifying cause of chronic arthritis, malabsorption, and increased skin pigmentation, I must consider Whipple's disease first and foremost. Physicians then were strapped and observation was often the default mode of the day. Given the abdominal findings, an exploratory laparotomy would be warranted if his condition deteriorated.

Despite forced oral feedings, the patient continued to lose weight, from his normal of 175 pounds to a nadir of 145 pounds. Because of worsening abdominal distention, the patient underwent exploratory abdominal surgery on the twenty-first hospital day. Intraoperatively, no ascites was seen, but his mesenteric lymph nodes were hard and markedly enlarged. The abdomen was closed without further intervention. Two days after the surgery, the patient abruptly developed dyspnea. His respirations were 40/minute, heart rate was 120, and he had minimal rales at the lung bases without findings of consolidation. He died 2 hours later, on the twenty-third hospital day, and an autopsy was performed.

The final event may have been a pulmonary embolism. As for the adenopathy, lymphoma and tuberculosis are possible. Heavy chain disease, an unusual lymphoproliferative disorder found in persons from the old Silk Trader's Route from the Middle East to the Orient, is a remote prospect. However, 5 years is just too indolent for most cancers and would be very unusual for tuberculosis. I think the findings support Whipple's disease, and I wonder if this was the first reported case.

On postmortem examination, the abdominal adenopathy was striking. The small intestine contained enlarged villi with thickened submucosa, and the mesenteric nodes were enlarged with fat deposits and abnormal "foamy cells." Within these foamy cells, microscopy revealed numerous rod-shaped organisms. All studies were negative for tuberculosis, and although the pathologist, Dr. George Hoyt Whipple, suspected an infectious etiology, he offered the name *intestinal lipodystrophy* to emphasize the striking small intestinal changes he witnessed at autopsy, which are the hallmarks of the disease that now bears his name. Whipple also shared the 1934 Nobel Prize in Physiology or Medicine with Minot and Murphy for their discovery that a nutritional substance in liver, now known as vitamin B12, was beneficial in treating pernicious anemia.

COMMENTARY

This is the index case of Whipple's disease, summarized from the original 1907 description.[1] George Hoyt Whipple, then a pathologist at Johns Hopkins, highlights the value of keen observation and a well-done case report in describing a new disease entity. One of the roles of case reports is to detail the features of an unknown disease. In this capacity, Whipple's summary is exemplary. His achievement was having the openness of mind to realize he was witnessing something novel and to take the first step on the road to discovery. Although Whipple suspected he was staring at a unique disease, he could not pinpoint the culprit bacteria and he had trouble squaring the extraintestinal findings with the marked intestinal anomalies. It was left to decades of input from others to confirm the association of arthralgias, eosinophilia, skin hyperpigmentation, and cardiac valve abnormalities with intestinal malabsorption and to culture the infectious agent.

In his discussion, Whipple recognized he was confronted with a novel clinical entity. Prior to surgery, pulmonary and mesenteric tuberculosis were suspected, based on the fevers, weight loss, cough, fat malabsorption, and lymphadenopathy. However, he felt the left apical exam was more representative of retraction from prior disease than active infection. He was also bothered by the negative skin reaction and sputum tests. At surgery, the pronounced adenopathy suggested sarcoma or Hodgkin's disease but postmortem examination eliminated these possibilities. At autopsy, the abdominal findings were most striking. The small intestine demonstrated enlarged villi with thickened submucosa and markedly enlarged mesenteric lymph glands containing large fat deposits and "distinctly abnormal foamy cells." These foamy macrophages contained "great numbers of rod-shaped organisms resembling the tubercle bacillus." However, all tests were negative for tuberculosis, and the lungs contained no active disease. Although he suspected an infectious etiology, Whipple offered the name *intestinal lipodystrophy* to emphasize the striking small intestinal pathology.

Although Whipple had surmised a novel infectious agent in 1907, it took almost a century to isolate the causative microbe. Granules within foamy macrophages of the small intestine were detected on periodic acid-Schiff (PAS) staining in 1949.[2] Similar PAS-positive granules were soon discovered in other tissues and fluid, providing a plausible explanation for the systemic features of the disease.[3] Electron microscopy confirmed the presence of infectious bacilli in 1961,[4] ushering in the era of antimicrobial treatment for this disease. More recently, using polymerase chain reaction (PCR), a unique bacterial 16S ribosomal RNA gene was isolated in patients with Whipple's disease.[5,6] Phylogenetically classified with the actinobacteria, *Tropheryma whipplei* (from the Greek *trophe*, nourishment, and *eryma*, barrier) was ultimately subcultured in 2000,[7] and immunodetection testing became possible. Using this technique, the archived pathology specimens from the 1907 index case demonstrated numerous intracellular bacteria in the lamina propria, closing the loop started by Whipple nearly a century earlier.[8]

Whipple's index case report described most of the manifestations of the disease we are familiar with today. As in the original description, arthralgias are the most common initial symptom and may precede diagnosis by a mean of 8 years. Other cardinal features include weight loss, abdominal pain, and steatorrhea due to small intestinal involvement. Table 7.1 summarizes the important signs and symptoms of Whipple's disease.[9,10] One notable manifestation missing in Whipple's report is central nervous system (CNS) involvement. CNS disease ranges from cognitive deficits to encephalitis and focal defects and may occur years after treatment and without concomitant intestinal symptoms.

A remaining mystery is why this pathogen results only rarely in clinical disease. Caucasians comprise the majority of infected patients, and men are affected eight times more often than women. An overrepresentation of HLA-B27 suggests a genetic predisposition; however, its role in pathogenesis is unclear. *T. whipplei* has been identified by PCR methods in asymptomatic individuals, implying additional abnormalities must be present in susceptible hosts for symptoms to occur following colonization.[11] The exact immune defects are speculative, and immunodeficiency states (such as HIV) have not been consistently identified in patients with Whipple's disease.

The cornerstone of diagnosing Whipple's disease is upper endoscopy with duodenal biopsy. Flattening of the villi and markedly increased PAS-positive staining of lamina propria macrophages are strongly suggestive of the diagnosis. However, PAS-positive staining is not unique to *T. whipplei*. In patients with profound immunodeficiency, *Mycobacterium avium intracellulare* may stain positive with PAS. Since Whipple's disease is only rarely associated with HIV, a negative HIV test would favor a diagnosis of Whipple's disease. Electron microscopy may distinguish *T. whipplei* from its mimickers by morphology. For extraintestinal disease, PCR testing on samples from infected tissue has been found to be a reliable diagnostic aid.[9]

TABLE 7.1 Clinical Features of Whipple's Disease

Clinical Feature	Comment
Cardinal Features (Present in 60%–90%)	
Arthropathy	Most common initial symptom, preceding diagnosis by a mean of 8 years Migratory, nonerosive, mainly in the peripheral joints
Weight loss	—
Diarrhea	Usually steatorrhea, may be associated with pain or occult blood in the stool
Other Common Features (Present in 20%–45%)	
Fever	—
Lymphadenopathy	May present as a palpable mass
Increased skin pigmentation	Mechanism unknown (evidence of adrenal insufficiency has not been found in Whipple's)
Cardiac disease	Culture-negative endocarditis
Hypotension	—
Peripheral edema	—
Uncommon Clinical Features	
Central nervous system involvement	May be global (dementia, personality change, sleep disturbance) or focal (cranial neuropathy, nystagmus)
Eye disease	Uveitis, retinitis
Hepatosplenomegaly	—
Polyserositis	—
Ascites	—

Two pathognomonic involuntary muscle signs in CNS Whipple's disease are oculomasticatory and oculofacial-skeletal myorhythmia.[10]

Given the rarity of the disease, controlled clinical trials addressing optimal treatment are lacking. Current recommendations include initial therapy for 14 days with an agent that crosses the blood–brain barrier (e.g., ceftriaxone) to reduce the incidence of CNS disease. This is then followed by a year or more of oral antimicrobial therapy with trimethoprim-sulfamethoxazole or a tetracycline.[9] While most patients respond within 2–3 weeks, relapse may occur in as many as one-third of patients.

Historical case reports reinforce the case-based learning paradigm. As the discussant remarks, observation was all too often the only recourse for physicians a century ago. In recounting the 7-year progression of the disease in one individual, Whipple provides a unique window into the natural evolution of the key features of this systemic disease. Viewed through the prism of Whipple's eyes, we can recall the striking lymphoid hyperplasia and unusual organisms in the small intestine, cementing our understanding of the pathogenesis of this disorder. Revisiting historical cases allows us to learn about, and also from, the past.

Key Points

1. Whipple's disease should be considered in patients with unexplained arthralgias accompanied by weight loss, malabsorption, and abdominal pain.
2. For suspected intestinal Whipple's disease, diagnosis is best made by duodenal biopsy demonstrating PAS-positive staining in lamina propria macrophages.

3. Less common systemic manifestations of Whipple's disease include culture-negative endocarditis and CNS disease. PCR testing of involved sites for *T. whipplei* is recommended to confirm extraintestinal disease.

REFERENCES

1. Whipple GH. A hitherto undescribed disease characterized anatomically by deposits of fat and fatty acids in the intestinal and mesenteric lymphatic tissues. *Bull Johns Hopkins Hosp*. 1907;18:382–391.
2. Black-Schaffer B. The tinctoral demonstration of a glycoprotein in Whipple's disease. *Proc Soc Exp Biol Med*. 1949;72:225–227.
3. Fleming JL, Wiesner RH, Shorter RG. Whipple's disease: clinical, biochemical, and histopathologic features and assessment of treatment in 29 patients. *Mayo Clin Proc*. 1988;63:539–551.
4. Yardley JH, Hendrix TR. Combined electron and light microscopy in Whipple's disease: demonstration of "bacillary bodies" in the intestine. *Bull Johns Hopkins Hosp*. 1961;109:80–98.
5. Wilson KH, Blitchington R, Frothingham R, Wilson JAP. Phylogeny of the Whipple's disease-associated bacterium. *Lancet*. 1991;338:474–475.
6. Relman DA, Schmidt TM, MacDermott RP, Falkow S. Identification of the uncultured bacillus of Whipple's disease. *N Engl J Med*. 1992;327:293–301.
7. Raoult D, Birg ML, La Scola B, et al. Cultivation of the bacillus of Whipple's disease. *N Engl J Med*. 2000;342:620–625.
8. Dumler SJ, Baisden BL, Yardley JH, Raoult D. Immunodetection of *Tropheryma whipplei* in intestinal tissue from Dr. Whipple's 1907 patient. *N Engl J Med*. 2003;348:1411–1412.
9. Marth T, Raoult D. Whipple's disease. *Lancet*. 2003;361:239–246.
10. Louis ED, Lynch T, Kaufmann P, et al. Diagnostic guidelines in central nervous system Whipple's disease. *Ann Neurol*. 1996;40:561–568.
11. Ehrbar HU, Bauerfeind P, Dutly F, et al. PCR-positive tests for *Tropheryma whipplei* in patients without Whipple's disease. *Lancet*. 1999;353:2214.

CHAPTER **8**

THE THIRD TIME'S THE CHARM

SARA MEKURIA
Internal Medicine Residency Program, Cleveland Clinic, Cleveland, Ohio

ESTEBAN CHENG CHING
Department of Neurology, Cleveland Clinic, Cleveland, Ohio

S. A. JOSEPHSON
Department of Neurology, University of California, San Francisco, California

JINNY TAVEE
Department of Neurology, Cleveland Clinic, Cleveland, Ohio

BRIAN J. HARTE
South Pointe Hospital, Cleveland Clinic Health System, Warrensville Heights, Ohio

A 58-year old woman was brought to the emergency department with confusion. Her husband stated that for several hours she had been "drifting in and out" at home and that he had to "shout to get her attention." He described no seizure activity, weakness, incontinence, or difficulty speaking and had noted no complaints of headache, fevers, chest pain, shortness of breath, or gastrointestinal complaints.

Altered mental status in a middle-aged woman can result from a diverse set of etiologies. A key distinction in the neurological examination will be to assure that the complaint of confusion is accurate as opposed to aphasia; the former is usually indicative of diffuse cerebral dysfunction, while the latter suggests a focal lesion in the dominant hemisphere.

The acuity of the change in mental status is important, as are the fluctuations described by the husband. Unwitnessed or nonconvulsive seizure activity can present this way. Toxic/metabolic etiologies, infectious and inflammatory disorders of the central nervous system (CNS), and vascular diseases are also important considerations. Although stroke does not typically present with global encephalopathy, intermittent large vessel occlusion, especially in the posterior circulation, can disrupt cognition in this manner. Following a physical examination, initial workup should focus on toxic/metabolic etiologies, followed rapidly by head imaging if no cause is identified.

Her past medical history was notable for type 2 diabetes mellitus, coronary artery disease, hyperlipidemia, and an unspecified seizure disorder, which, according to her husband, was diagnosed during a recent hospitalization for a similar presentation. She also had a remote history of venous thromboembolism and antithrombin III deficiency. She was unemployed, lived with her husband, and spent most of

Clinical Care Conundrums: Challenging Diagnoses in Hospital Medicine, First Edition.
Edited by James C. Pile, Thomas E. Baudendistel, and Brian J. Harte.

her time at home. She never smoked and rarely drank alcohol. Her family history was unobtainable, and her husband denied that she used any illicit drugs. Her medications included pioglitazone, aspirin, simvastatin, pregabalin, ferrous sulfate, levetiracetam, warfarin, and magnesium oxide, and she was allergic to sulfa.

While the differential diagnosis remains broad, three elements of the history are potentially relevant. The history of epilepsy based on a similar prior presentation increases the likelihood that the current spell is ictal in nature; examination of previous records would be important in order to document whether these spells have indeed been proven to be epileptic, as many conditions can mimic seizures. Given the history of venous thromboembolism and hypercoagulability, one must consider cerebral venous sinus thrombosis, which can present with global neurologic dysfunction and seizures. Prompt identification, usually via computed tomography (CT) or magnetic resonance angiography, is vital because anticoagulation can mitigate this potentially life-threatening illness. Finally, although many medications can cause encephalopathy in overdose, levetiracetam has well-described cognitive side effects even at usual doses, including encephalopathy, irritability, and depression.

The records from that recent hospitalization remarked that she had presented confused and "stuporous." Her potassium had been 2.7 mmol/L; international normalized ratio (INR), 3.4; and hemoglobin, 8 g/dL; other routine laboratory studies were normal. CT and magnetic resonance imaging (MRI) of the brain had been negative, and electroencephalogram (EEG) reportedly was performed but specific results were unknown. She was discharged alert and oriented 1 week prior to the current presentation on the above medications, including levetiracetam for this newly diagnosed "seizure disorder."

Previous records confirm that the current presentation is that of a relapsing acute alteration in mental status. Regardless of the EEG findings or response to antiepileptic medications, a seizure disorder should remain a primary consideration, although relapsing inflammatory, toxic/metabolic conditions, and, rarely, vascular disorders can also present in this manner.

The neurologic manifestations of hypokalemia are usually peripheral in nature, including periodic paralysis; confusion accompanying hypokalemia is usually not a result of the low potassium itself but rather due to an underlying toxic or endocrinologic cause. Various causes of anemia can lead to mental status changes; the mean corpuscular volume (MCV) will be particularly helpful given known associations between megaloblastic anemia and confusional states.

On examination, she appeared to be in good health and in no distress. She was afebrile. Her blood pressure was 93/57; pulse, 90 beats per minute; respiratory rate, 16/minute; and room air oxygen saturation, 100%. She was oriented to her surroundings, but slow in her responses to questioning. There were no cranial nerve, motor, or sensory deficits, or abnormal reflexes or movements. Examination of the head, skin, chest, cardiovascular system, abdomen, and extremities was normal. Serum sodium was 136 mmol/L; creatinine, 1.2 mg/dL; calcium, 9.3 mg/dL; and glucose, 81 mg/dL; other routine blood chemistries were normal. Her white blood cell (WBC) count was 7100/μL, hemoglobin was 9.2 g/dL with normal MCV, and platelet count was 275,000/μL. INR was 3.4, and liver function tests were normal. CT of the brain demonstrated no evidence of acute pathology.

Given that her laboratory results (aside from the hemoglobin) and CT were essentially normal, the most common etiology of a recurrent encephalopathy would be a toxic exposure including drugs, alcohol, and environmental toxins or poisons. A comprehensive serum drug screen, including heavy metals, could follow a basic urinary screen for drugs of abuse; specific etiologies may be suggested by patterns of injury seen on MRI, such as those seen with carbon monoxide or methanol exposure. Other recurrent metabolic processes include porphyrias and relapsing inflammatory disorders, which could be entertained if further diagnostics are unrevealing.

An EEG is warranted at this point and is a test that is underutilized in the workup of altered mental status. Patients who have a spell and do not quickly awaken should be considered to be in nonconvulsive status epilepticus until proven otherwise. This can be easily identified on the EEG and is an important entity to recognize quickly. Additional findings on EEG may suggest focal cerebral dysfunction (such as that following a seizure or acute unilateral injury), diffuse encephalopathy (e.g., triphasic waves), or fairly specific diagnoses (e.g., periodic lateralized epileptiform discharges from the temporal lobes in suspected herpes simplex meningoencephalitis). While the CT of the brain is a reasonable initial screen, MRI is more sensitive for structural disease and should be obtained if no etiology is rapidly identified.

Finally, acute infectious etiologies such as abscess, encephalitis, or meningoencephalitis need to be excluded via lumbar puncture. Spinal fluid examination can also be helpful in the consideration of inflammatory and autoimmune disorders.

Over the next several hours, while still in the emergency department, she became increasingly obtunded, to the point that she was unresponsive to all stimuli. No seizure activity was witnessed, her vital signs were unchanged, and no medications had been administered. She was urgently transferred to a tertiary care center, where, at the time of arrival, she was obtunded and nonverbal, and opened her eyes only to noxious stimuli. She would withdraw all four extremities in response to pain. Pupils were 2 mm and symmetrically reactive. Corneal reflexes were normal, and her gag reflex was diminished. Motor tone was decreased in all 4 extremities. No fasciculations were noted. Deep tendon reflexes were present but symmetrically diminished throughout, and the Babinski testing demonstrated a withdrawal response bilaterally.

Coma is a state of profound unconsciousness where the patient is unarousable and unaware of his or her surroundings. Coma can result either from bihemispheric dysfunction or diffuse injury to the reticular activating system in the brainstem, and the physical examination should focus on distinguishing between these two sites. Because the nuclei of cranial nerves III through XII (excepting XI) reside in the brainstem, the coma examination emphasizes on testing the cranial nerves; although all cranial nerves are not tested in this patient, the ones tested appear to be normal, making bihemispheric dysfunction most likely. Bihemispheric coma most commonly results from diffuse toxic or metabolic etiologies such as intoxication or hepatic encephalopathy, but it can also be caused by bilateral structural lesions (including the bilateral thalami) or ongoing seizure activity.

Although an EEG remains the key test in this patient and an MRI would be extremely useful, her deterioration warrants a workup for CNS infection. Since the head CT was negative, it would be prudent to proceed with urgent lumbar puncture (although it should never be performed in a patient with significant coagulopathy due to risks of hemorrhage leading to spinal cord injury). She should be covered empirically with broad-spectrum meningeal-dose antibiotics, including acyclovir, until the results of the spinal fluid examination are known, given that bacterial meningitis and herpes meningoencephalitis carry a high morbidity and mortality if not treated promptly.

Routine blood tests were similar to her labs at the referring emergency room. Ammonia level was 10 μmol/L. Urine toxicology screen was negative, and blood tests for ethanol, salicylates, lithium, and acetaminophen were negative. Chest X-ray and urinalysis were normal, and electrocardiogram was notable only for a sinus tachycardia. Cultures of the blood were obtained, and the patient was admitted to the intensive care unit.

Levetiracetam, vancomycin, piperacillin-tazobactam, and acyclovir were initiated. A lumbar puncture was performed without reversing the anticoagulation, and the procedure was traumatic. The cerebrospinal fluid (CSF) was bloody, with a clear supernatant. Cell count demonstrated a red blood cell (RBC) count of 1250/μL and a WBC count of 9/μL, with a WBC differential of 42% neutrophils, 48% lymphocytes, and 8% monocytes. The CSF glucose was 62 mg/dL (with a serum glucose of 74 mg/dL) and protein was 41 mg/dL. The CSF Gram stain demonstrated no organisms, and fluid was sent for routine culture and polymerase chain reaction (PCR) to detect herpes simplex virus (HSV). A neurology consultation was urgently requested.

As mentioned, it would have been more appropriate to reverse the patient's anticoagulation prior to lumbar puncture. The absence of xanthochromia suggests that the RBCs seen in the sample were introduced at the time of the lumbar puncture, arguing against a hemorrhagic disorder of the CNS (occasionally seen with herpes simplex encephalitis) or spinal fluid (e.g., subarachnoid hemorrhage).

A reasonable rule of thumb to correct for the number of RBCs in a traumatic lumbar puncture is to allow 1 WBC for every 700 RBCs/μL. Given this conversion, there are still too many WBCs in this sample, indicating a mild pleocytosis that is approximately one-half neutrophilic and one-half lymphocytic. This profile is nonspecific and can occur with a variety of conditions including stroke, seizure, inflammatory disorders, and infections, including viruses such as West Nile virus.

While coverage with acyclovir and broad-spectrum antibacterials is appropriate, it should be noted that piperacillin-tazobactam has poor CSF penetration and therefore is not a good choice for empiric coverage of CNS infections.

The neurologist's examination additionally noted "multifocal myoclonus with noxious stimuli, most prominent in the face and toes." An urgent EEG demonstrated continuous, slow, generalized triphasic wave activity (Figs. 8.1 and 8.2); no epileptiform discharges were seen. The erythrocyte sedimentation rate (ESR) was 66 mm/hour (normal, 0–30), and tests for antinuclear antibodies, serum levetiracetam level, and thyroid function studies were ordered.

Stimulus-evoked multifocal myoclonus is a general marker of encephalopathy found in many conditions, including hepatic and renal failure, drug intoxication (e.g., opiates), neurodegenerative disorders (e.g., Creutzfeldt–Jakob disease [CJD]), and postanoxic injury, the latter of which is termed the *Lance–Adams syndrome*.

Triphasic waves on EEG, while commonly associated with hepatic encephalopathy, have a similarly broad differential diagnosis, although in a comatose patient, they must first and foremost be distinguished from the repetitive discharges characteristic of nonconvulsive status epilepticus. In addition to hepatic and renal failure, triphasic waves have also been described in medication toxicity (especially with anticonvulsants, lithium, and cephalosporins), CNS infections (including Lyme disease and West Nile virus

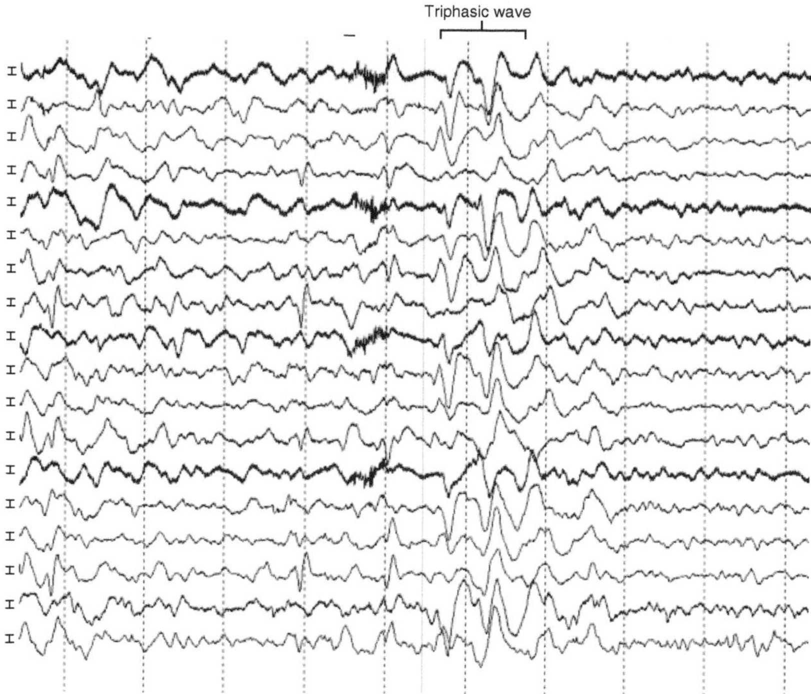

FIGURE 8.1 Patient's EEG, demonstrating triphasic waves, which are characterized by an initial negative wave (upward), followed by a deep positivity (downward) and then a negative wave, superimposed on diffuse slowing. **Abbreviation**: EEG, electroencephalogram.

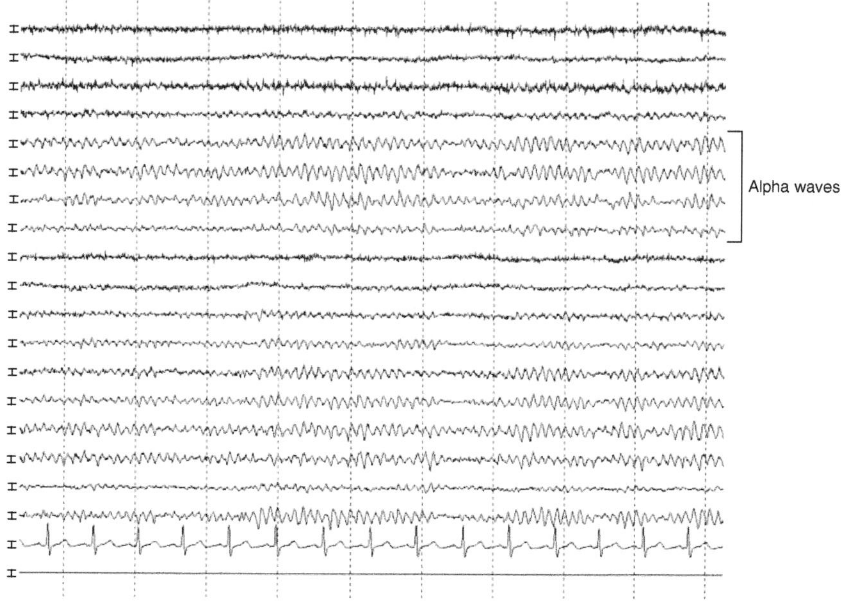

FIGURE 8.2 Normal EEG of another patient with characteristic alpha waves of 8–9 Hz in the background. **Abbreviation**: EEG, electroencephalogram.

infection), strokes involving the bilateral thalami (usually from deep venous thrombosis), inflammatory disorders (such as Hashimoto's encephalopathy [HE]), and neurodegenerative diseases. It is important to remember that a single EEG does not exclude the possibility of an episodic ictal disorder and longer-term monitoring would be required to definitively exclude seizures.

At this point, although the myoclonus and triphasic waves most commonly would indicate a toxic/metabolic process, the elevated ESR and CSF pleocytosis argue for an inflammatory or infectious condition. An MRI remains the next most useful test to guide further workup because many such conditions have distinct signatures on MRI.

The following day, she was noted to have periods of alertness—opening her eyes and following some commands—but at other times, she was difficult to arouse or obtunded. Tremulous movements and sporadic myoclonic jerks continued but no focal neurologic signs were found. Although there was increased muscle tone throughout, she was intermittently seen moving her limbs spontaneously, but not to command. No new findings were appreciated on routine laboratory tests. Antinuclear antibody testing was negative. Serum levetiracetam level was 23.5 μg/mL (reference range, 5–45). Serum thyroid-stimulating hormone was less than 0.005 μU/mL, but free T3 was 3.5 pg/mL (normal, 1.8–4.6) and free T4 was 2.0 ng/dL (normal, 0.7–1.8). An MRI of the brain was compromised by motion artifact but no significant abnormalities were appreciated.

At this point, a family member in another state disclosed that the patient had also been hospitalized 2 months previously while visiting him. Her chief complaint had been shortness of breath. The records were obtained; a cardiac catheterization had revealed nonobstructive coronary disease, and medical management was recommended. The notes mentioned that during the hospitalization she developed "altered mental status with disorientation and shaking." CT and MRI of the brain had been unremarkable. The confusion was not explained, but she was discharged in good condition, alert and fully oriented.

The additional history confirms a relapsing encephalopathy, now with at least three occurrences. The most common etiologies in the face of a normal MRI and basic labs would be recurrent intoxication or exposures, but the inflammatory CSF profile and elevated ESR are not consistent with this. A variety of inflammatory disorders can present with recurrent encephalopathy, including demyelinating diseases and neurosarcoidosis. Some systemic rheumatologic conditions, such as systemic lupus erythematosus, can present with relapsing neurologic symptoms due to seizures, vasculitis, or cerebritis. Vasculitis would fit this picture as well, except for the normal findings on two MRIs. In a patient with such dramatic symptoms of neurologic dysfunction, one would expect to see changes on the MRI of cerebral inflammation with probable ischemia.

Therefore, given the CSF, ESR, clinical course, and unrevealing MRI and EEG, the most likely group of disorders responsible would be the nonvasculitic autoimmune meningoencephalitides, which present with recurrent encephalopathy and feature spontaneous remissions and/or often-dramatic responses to corticosteroids. Key disorders in this category include Sjogren's disease, lupus, and steroid-responsive encephalopathy associated with autoimmune thyroiditis (HE). Steroid-responsive encephalopathy is the most common of the group and is suggested by the abnormal thyroid-stimulating hormone testing, although it may occur in the setting of normal thyroid function. The diagnosis can be confirmed with thyroperoxidase and thyroglobulin antibody testing.

Three days into hospitalization, her mental status had gradually improved such that she was more consistently awake and oriented to person and place, and she was transferred to a regular nursing unit. Final results from the CSF and blood cultures were negative, as was PCR for HSV. The antimicrobials were discontinued. Routine serum chemistries continued to be unremarkable. Additional studies recommended by the neurologist demonstrated an antithyroperoxidase antibody concentration of 587.1 IU/mL (normal, <5), and antithyroglobulin antibody level of 52.2 IU/mL (normal, <10).

These results confirm the diagnosis of HE that, in addition to its presentation as a recurrent illness, is an important treatable cause of dementia and should be considered in young patients, those with autoimmune and thyroid disorders, and those whose dementia is rapidly progressive. Most cases are thought to be steroid responsive, but some studies have defined the disorder based on this responsiveness, resulting in some nonresponders likely being overlooked.

A trial of corticosteroids should be considered if the patient does not quickly return to baseline, given the potential morbidities associated with prolonged altered mental status to this degree. Whether initiation of chronic immunosuppression could prevent these attacks in the future is unclear from the literature but should be considered given the recurrent, dramatic presentation in this patient.

A diagnosis of HE was made, and she was prescribed corticosteroids. Twenty-four hours later, she was alert and fully oriented. She was discharged to home on prednisone and seen in follow-up in neurology clinic 1 month later. She had had no further episodes of confusion or stupor, but because of steroid-induced hyperglycemia, her corticosteroids were decreased and mycophenolate mofetil was added for chronic immunosuppression. Four months after discharge, she was neurologically stable but continued to struggle with the adverse effects of chronic corticosteroid treatment.

COMMENTARY

HE is an uncommon condition that can present with a rapidly progressive decline and should be considered in patients who present with recurrent mental status changes in the setting of normal imaging studies and routine laboratory results. The entity was initially described by Lord William Russell Brain in 1966 and in the most recent terminology is known as *steroid-responsive encephalopathy associated with autoimmune thyroiditis* (*SREAT*).[1] It is characterized by an acute or subacute encephalopathy associated with thyroid autoimmunity. Patients typically present with fluctuating symptoms, episodes of confusion, alterations of consciousness, and rapid cognitive decline.[2] Common features include myoclonus, tremor, ataxia, speech disturbance, stroke-like episodes, increased muscle tone, neuropsychiatric manifestations, and seizures that, in some cases, may progress to status epilepticus.[3,4]

Although serum antithyroglobulin and antithyroperoxidase antibodies are elevated in HE, their presence is thought to be an epiphenomenon of the condition rather than the direct cause. Supporting this are the facts that the incidence of encephalopathy is not increased in patients with established autoimmune thyroiditis, and the presence of antithyroid antibodies ranges from 5% to 20% in the general population.[2,5] There is also no evidence that thyroid antibodies directly react with brain tissue, and the levels of these antibodies do not correlate with either neurologic manifestations or clinical improvement.[2,4,5] As HE has been reported in patients with euthyroidism, hypothyroidism, and hyperthyroidism (with hypothyroidism—either subclinical or active—most common), it is also unlikely that the level of thyroid hormones play a role in the etiology of this disease.[2,4,6]

The etiology and pathogenesis of HE are unclear, although an immune-mediated process is generally implicated, either from an inflammatory vasculitis or as a form of acute disseminated encephalomyelitis.[7–9] Global hypoperfusion on single-photon emission computed tomography (SPECT) studies has also been reported.[10,11] Patients with HE may have nonspecific evidence of inflammation, including an elevated ESR, CRP, and CSF protein.[12] Other laboratory abnormalities may include a mild elevation of liver aminotransferase levels; renal impairment has also been reported in a few cases of HE in the form of glomerulonephritis and may be related to deposition of immune complexes containing thyroglobulin antigen.[6,12–14] MRI of the brain is normal or nonspecific in most cases, and the EEG most commonly shows diffuse slowing.

The differential for a rapidly progressive cognitive decline includes CJD, CNS vasculitis, paraneoplastic syndromes, and autoimmune and subacute infectious encephalopathies. In patients with CJD, T2-weighted imaging may show hyperintense signals in the basal ganglia, while diffusion-weighted sequences may reveal changes in the cortical ribbon and bilateral thalami.[15] In CNS vasculitis, the imaging findings are variable and range from discrete areas of vascular infarcts to hemorrhagic lesions.[16] In paraneoplastic and autoimmune encephalopathies (excluding HE), MRI often shows nonenhancing signal intensity changes in the mesial temporal lobes.[12] This patient had repeatedly normal MRI studies of the brain, which in combination with the history of tremor, myoclonus, seizures, and interval return to baseline status helped point to the diagnosis of HE.

Different approaches to the treatment of HE have been recommended. As the acronym SREAT suggests, patients typically respond dramatically to high-dose steroid therapy. Although a number of patients also improve spontaneously, up to 60% of patients experience a relapsing course and require chronic immunosuppressive agents for maintenance therapy, including long-term steroids and azathioprine.[2,17] Treatment with plasma exchange and intravenous immunoglobulin has also been reported, but with mixed results.[18,19] Due to her history of multiple relapses, the patient was placed on mycophenolate mofetil for additional maintenance immunosuppression, as her corticosteroid dose was reduced due to adverse effects.

Acute mental status change is a potentially emergent situation that must be evaluated with careful history and studies to exclude life-threatening metabolic, infectious, and vascular conditions. This patient presented similarly on two prior occasions, and each time her physician team evaluated what appeared to be a new onset of altered consciousness, reaching a plausible but ultimately incorrect diagnosis. The patient's third presentation was finally the charm, as her physicians learned of the repeated history of a confusional state and, in particular, the return to baseline status, allowing them to create a differential that focused on etiologies of relapsing encephalopathy and to make the correct diagnosis.

Key Points

1. *Recurrent* acute or subacute cognitive deterioration invokes a differential diagnosis of toxic/metabolic disorders and unusual inflammatory conditions.

2. The nonvasculitic autoimmune encephalopathies are a group of uncommon conditions characterized by nonspecific findings of inflammation and generally unremarkable CNS imaging studies.
3. HE or SREAT, is the most common of these conditions and is notable for mental status changes, various findings of increased muscular tone, thyroid autoimmunity, and, generally, a dramatic response to corticosteroids.

REFERENCES

1. Brain LWR, Jellinek EH, Ball K. Hashimoto's disease and encephalopathy. *Lancet*. 1966;2:512–514.
2. Chong JY, Rowland LP, Utiger RD. Hashimoto encephalopathy: syndrome or myth? *Arch Neurol*. 2003;60:164–171.
3. Ferlazzo E, Raffaele M, Mazzu I, Pisani F. Recurrent status epilepticus as the main feature of Hashimoto's encephalopathy. *Epilepsy Behav*. 2006;8:328–330.
4. Castillo P, Woodruff B, Caselli R, et al. Steroid-responsive encephalopathy associated with autoimmune thyroiditis. *Arch Neurol*. 2006;63:197–202.
5. Kothbauer-Margreiter I, Sturznegger M, Komor J, Baumgartner R, Hess C. Encephalopathy associated with Hashimoto thyroiditis: diagnosis and treatment. *J Neurol*. 1996;243:585–593.
6. Shaw PJ, Walls TJ, Newman PK, Cleland PG, Cartlidge NE. Hashimoto's encephalopathy: a steroid-responsive disorder associated with high antithyroid antibody titers-report of 5 cases. *Neurology*. 1991;41:228–233.
7. Nolte KW, Unbehaun A, Sieker H, Kloss TM, Paulus W. Hashimoto encephalopathy: a brainstem vasculitis? *Neurology*. 2000;54:769–770.
8. Caselli RJ, Boeve BF, Scheithauer BW, O'Duffy JD, Hunder GG. Nonvasculitic autoimmune inflammatory meningoencephalitis (NAIM): A reversible form of encephalopathy. *Neurology*. 1999;53:1579–1581.
9. Duffey P, Yee S, Reid IN, Bridges LR. Hashimoto's encephalopathy: postmortem findings after fatal status epilepticus. *Neurology*. 2003;61:1124–1126.
10. Forchetti CM, Katsamakis G, Garron DC. Autoimmune thyroiditis and a rapidly progressive dementia: global hypoperfusion on SPECT scanning suggests a possible mechanism. *Neurology*. 1997;49:623–626.
11. Kalita J, Misra UK, Rathore C, Pradhan PK, Das BK. Hashimoto's encephalopathy: clinical, SPECT and neurophysiologic data. *QJM*. 2003;96:455–457.
12. Vernino S, Geschwind M, Bradley B. Autoimmune encephalopathies. *Neurologist*. 2007;13:140–147.
13. O'Regan S, Fong JSC, Kaplan BS, De Chadarevian JP, Lapointe N, Drummond KN. Thyroid antigen-antibody nephritis. *Clin Immunol Immunopathol*. 1976;6:341–346.
14. Jordan SC, Johnston WH, Bergstein JM. Immune complex glomerulonephritis mediated by thyroid antigens. *Arch Pathol Lab Med*. 1978;102:530–533.
15. Ukisu R, Kushihashi T, Tanaka E, et al. Diffusion-weighted MR imaging of early-stage Creutzfeldt-Jakob disease: Typical and atypical manifestations. *RadioGraphics*. 2006;26:S191–S204.
16. Pomper MG, Miller TJ, Stone JH, Tidmore WC, Hellmann DB. CNS vasculitis in autoimmune disease: MR imaging findings and correlation with angiography. *AJNR Am J Neuroradiol*. 1999;20:75–85.
17. Marshal GA, Doyle JJ. Long-term treatment of Hashimoto's encephalopathy. *J Neuropsychiatry Clin Neurosci*. 2006;18:14–20.
18. Jacob S, Rajabally YA. Hashimoto's encephalopathy: steroid resistance and response to intravenouc immunoglobulins. *J Neurol Neurosurg Psychiatry*. 2005;76:455–456.
19. Boers PM, Colebatch JG. Hashimoto's encephalopathy responding to plasmapheresis. *J Neurol Neurosurg Psychiatry*. 2001;70:132.

CHAPTER 9

A FRAYED KNOT

THOMAS E. BAUDENDISTEL
Department of Medicine, Kaiser Permanente Medical Center, Oakland, California

IRENA L. ILIC
Department of Medicine, Palo Alto Medical Foundation, Palo Alto, California

HARRY HOLLANDER
Department of Medicine, University of California, San Francisco, California

A 20-year-old woman presented to the emergency department after 2 days of epistaxis and vaginal bleeding.

A young woman is more likely to present with infection, toxic exposure, or rheumatologic disease than with a degenerative disease or malignancy. Her bleeding may relate to a platelet abnormality, either quantitative or qualitative. I would pursue her bleeding and menstrual history further.

The patient was healthy until 2 months previously, when she noted arthralgia of her shoulders, wrists, elbows, knees, and ankles. She was examined by a rheumatologist who detected mild arthritis in her left wrist and proximal interphalangeal joints. The rest of her joints were normal. Rheumatoid factor and antinuclear antibody (ANA) were positive, and the erythrocyte sedimentation rate was 122 mm/hour. She was diagnosed with possible systemic lupus erythematosus (SLE) and was placed on a nonsteroidal anti-inflammatory agent. At a follow-up visit 1 month prior to admission, her arthralgias had markedly improved. Two weeks prior to admission, the patient began to feel fatigued. Two days prior to admission, she developed epistaxis and what she thought was her menses, although bleeding was heavier than usual and associated with the passage of red clots. On the day of admission, the vaginal bleeding worsened and emergency personnel transported the patient to the hospital.

Securing a diagnosis of SLE can be challenging. One must be vigilant for other diseases masquerading as SLE while continuing to build a case for it. As more criteria are fulfilled, the probability of lupus increases, yet no findings, alone or in combination, are pathognomonic of this protean disease. This patient's age, sex, and serology are compatible with SLE; otherwise, her presentation is nonspecific. I would request a complete blood count, coagulation tests, and additional serological tests.

The quantity of the bleeding is described, but this does not help decipher its etiology. Excess bleeding may be a result of one or more of three broad etiologies: problems with platelets (quantitative or qualitative), with clotting factors (quantitative

---

Clinical Care Conundrums: Challenging Diagnoses in Hospital Medicine, First Edition.
Edited by James C. Pile, Thomas E. Baudendistel, and Brian J. Harte.

or qualitative), or with blood vessels (trauma, vasculitis, or diseases affecting collagen). Because quantitative and qualitative factor disorders generally do not present with mucosal bleeding, platelet disorders, and vascular problems are of greater concern. If this woman has lupus, immunologic thrombocytopenia may be the cause of mucosal bleeding.

The patient had no previous medical problems and had never been pregnant. Her only medication was sulindac twice daily for the past month. She was born in Hong Kong, graduated from high school in San Francisco, and attended junior college. She lived with her parents and brother and denied alcohol, tobacco, or recreational drug use but had recently obtained a tattoo on her lower back. There was no family history of autoimmune or bleeding disorders, and a review of systems was notable for dyspnea with minimal exertion and fatigue that worsened in the past 2 days. She had no prior episodes of abnormal bleeding or clotting.

Tattoos may be surrogates for other high-risk behaviors and suggest an increased risk of hepatitis and sexually transmitted diseases. Her sexual history and other risk factors for human immunodeficiency virus infection must be investigated. The dyspnea and fatigue are likely the result of anemia, although it is too early to rule out cardiac or pulmonary disease.

On arrival at the emergency department, the patient had a blood pressure of 78/46 mm Hg, a pulse of 120 beats per minute, a temperature of 34°C, 14 respirations per minute, and oxygen saturation of 99% while breathing supplemental oxygen through a nonrebreather mask. Systolic blood pressure improved to 90 mm Hg after 4 L of normal saline was administered. The patient was pale but alert. There was crusted blood in her mouth and nostrils without active bleeding or petechiae. Her tongue was pierced with a ring, and sclerae were anicteric. Bleeding was noted from both nipples. There was no heart murmur or gallop, and jugular venous pressure was not elevated. Pulmonary exam revealed bibasilar crackles. Abdomen was soft, not tender, and without hepatosplenomegaly, and her umbilicus was pierced by a ring. Genitourinary exam revealed scant vaginal discharge and clotted blood in the vagina. Skin demonstrated no petechiae, ecchymoses, or stigmata of liver disease. Neurological and joint exams were normal.

It is hard to conceive of vaginal bleeding producing this profound a degree of hypotension. The patient may have additional occult sites of bleeding, or she may have a distributive cause of hypotension, such as sepsis or adrenal hemorrhage with resultant adrenal insufficiency. Breast bleeding is unusual, even with profound thrombocytopenia, and raises the possibility of a concomitant factor deficiency. Furthermore, if thrombocytopenia were the sole reason for the bleeding, petechiae should be present. Diffuse vascular injury, such as from lupus or vasculitis, would be an unusual cause of profound bleeding unless there was also disseminated intravascular coagulation.

Laboratory studies revealed a white count of 2000/mm^3, of which 42% were neutrophils, 40% bands, 8% lymphocytes, and 10% monocytes. Hematocrit was 17.6% and platelets were 35,000/mm^3. Sodium was 124 mmol/L; potassium, 6 mmol/L; chloride, 92 mmol/L; bicarbonate, 10 mmol/L; blood urea nitrogen, 122 mg/dL (43.5 mmol/L); and creatinine, 3.4 mg/dL (300 μmol/L). Blood glucose was 44 mg/dL (2.44 mmol/L). Total bilirubin was 3.0 mg/dL (51.3 μmol/L; normal range, 0.1–1.5); alkaline phosphatase, 105 U/L (normal range, 39–117); aspartate aminotransferase, 849 U/L (normal range, 8–31); alanine aminotransferase, 261 U/L (normal range, 7–31); international normalized unit (INR), 2.9; and partial thromboplastin time (PTT) 34.2 seconds.

The combination of profound hypotension, electrolyte abnormalities, hypoglycemia, and hypothermia makes adrenal insufficiency a consideration. I would perform a cosyntropin stimulation test and start glucocorticoid and perhaps mineralocorticoid replacement. In addition, there is renal failure and metabolic acidosis, with a calculated anion gap of 22. The anion gap may be from lactic acidosis secondary to hypotension and hypoperfusion. The abnormal transaminases and bilirubin could relate to infectious hepatitis or systemic infection. Although ischemia could explain these findings, it is rare for a 20 year old to develop ischemic hepatopathy. Thrombocytopenia may contribute to the volume of blood loss, but spontaneous bleeding because of thrombocytopenia is unusual until the platelet count falls below 20,000/mm^3. Furthermore, the elevated INR points to a mixed coagulopathy. This is not the pattern seen with antiphospholipid antibody syndrome, in which the INR tends to be preserved and the PTT prolonged. Interpretation of the INR is complicated by the fact that she has liver disease, and of highest concern is the possibility of acute disseminated intravascular coagulation (DIC) or impending fulminant hepatic failure.

Urine dipstick testing demonstrated a specific gravity of 1.015, trace leukocyte esterase, 2+ protein, and 3+ blood, and microscopy revealed 2 white blood cells and 38 red blood cells per high-power field, many bacteria, and no casts. Creatine kinase was 20,599 U/L, with a myocardial fraction of 1.4%. Lipase was normal, lactate was 7.3 mmol/L, and serum pregnancy test was negative.

Although there is proteinuria and hematuria, there is no solid evidence of glomerulonephritis. I would examine her sediment carefully for dysmorphic red cells, recognizing that only a quarter of people with glomerulonephritis have red-cell casts. A urine protein-to-creatinine ratio would be useful for estimating the degree of proteinuria. The elevated creatine kinase indicates rhabdomyolysis. In a previously healthy young woman without evidence of cardiogenic shock, it would be unusual for hypotension to result in rhabdomyolysis. Infection and metabolic derangements are possible etiologies of rhabdomyolysis. Alternatively, coagulopathy might have produced intramuscular bleeding. The constellation of thrombocytopenia, anemia, and renal failure raises my suspicion that there is a thrombotic microangiopathy, such as thrombotic thrombocytopenic purpura (TTP) or hemolytic uremic syndrome (HUS). I would inspect a peripheral-blood smear for schistocytes and evidence of microangiopathy.

The chest radiograph demonstrated low lung volumes, patchy areas of consolidation, and pulmonary edema. Heart size was normal, and there were no pleural effusions. On the first hospital day the patient required mechanical ventilation because of respiratory failure. She received 5 units of packed red blood cells, 2 units of fresh frozen plasma, and 1 unit of platelets. Vasopressor infusion was started, and a vascular catheter was placed for hemodialysis. Blood, respiratory, and urine cultures were sent, and methylprednisolone, piperacillin/tazobactam, and vancomycin were administered. D-dimer was greater than 10,000 ng/mL, fibrinogen was 178 mg/dL, and lactate dehydrogenase was 1671 U/L. The peripheral-blood smear demonstrated 1+ schistocytes and no spherocytes.

The presence of schistocytes and the elevated lactate dehydrogenase point to a microangiopathic hemolytic process. Causes of microangiopathic hemolytic anemia include TTP, HUS, DIC, paraneoplastic conditions, and endothelial damage from malignant hypertension or scleroderma renal crisis. The INR and PTT will usually be normal in TTP and HUS. The depressed fibrinogen and elevated D-dimer suggest that in response to severe bleeding, she is also clotting. DIC, possibly from a severe infection, would explain these findings. Alternatively, the multisystem organ failure may represent progression of SLE.

Additional serology studies detected antinuclear antibodies at 1:320, with a speckled pattern. Rheumatoid factor was not present, but anti-double-stranded DNA and anti-Smith antibodies were elevated. C3 was 30 mg/dL (normal range, 90–180), C4 was 24 mg/dL (normal range, 16–47), and the erythrocyte sedimentation rate was 53 mm/hour.

The results of the additional lab tests support a diagnosis of lupus and thus a lupus flare, but I agree that antibiotics should be empirically administered while searching for an underlying infection that might mimic lupus. Apart from infection, severe lupus may be complicated by widespread vasculitis or catastrophic antiphospholipid antibody syndrome, which would necessitate high-dose immunosuppressive therapy and anticoagulation, respectively.

Tests for antiphospholipid antibodies including lupus anticoagulant and for anticardiolipin antibodies were negative. The patient continued to require vasopressors, hemodialysis, and mechanical ventilation. On the fourth hospital day, she developed a morbilliform rash over her trunk, face, and extremities. Skin over her right buttock became indurated and tender. On the sixth day of hospitalization, the skin on her face, extremities, and palms began to desquamate (Fig. 9.1).

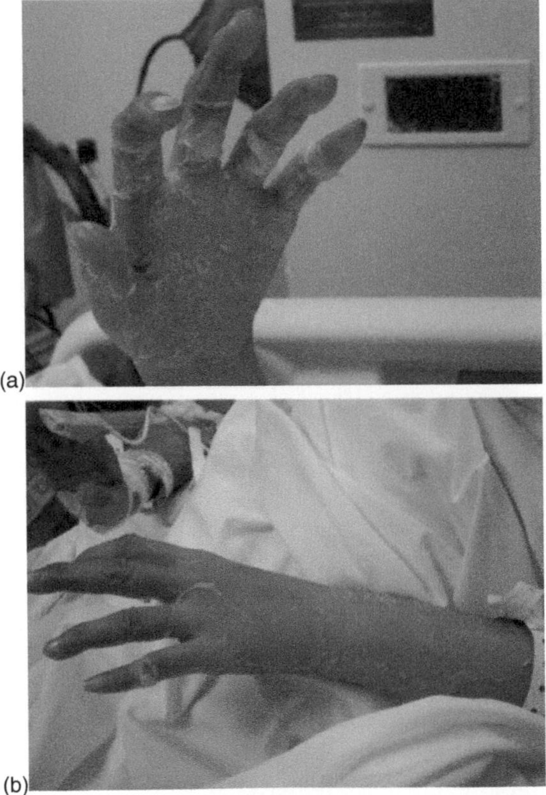

FIGURE 9.1 Photographic images from hospital day 6: (a) desquamating, degloving hand rash and (b) desquamating, degloving hand rash extending onto the dorsum of the arm.

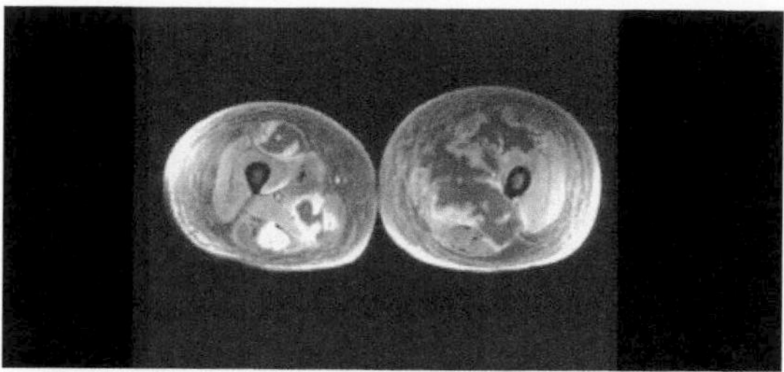

FIGURE 9.2 T1-weighted MRI (with fat saturation) of the thighs. There is extensive liquefactive necrosis involving multiple thigh muscles that is greater in the left thigh than the right thigh.

Regarding the rash, it is hard to differentiate the chicken from the egg. The rash may be a reaction to medication, a clue to a multiorgan disease, or a manifestation of severe skin reactions, such as Stevens–Johnson syndrome, as well as bacterial toxin-mediated diseases, such as toxic shock syndrome (TSS). The criteria for TSS with multisystem involvement are very similar to those for lupus. In this case, a desquamating rash occurring on the heel of a multiorgan illness definitely points to TSS. In staphylococcal toxic shock cases, blood cultures are frequently negative, and the origin may elude detection, but of the sources identified, most have been wounds and soft tissue infections.

On hospital day 4, blood cultures from admission grew oxacillin-sensitive *Staphylococcus aureus* in four of the four bottles. Magnetic resonance imaging of the thigh demonstrated extensive necrosis of multiple muscles (Fig. 9.2). The patient underwent muscle debridement in the operating room, and Gram's stain of the debrided muscle revealed Gram-positive cocci. Following surgery, she rapidly improved. She no longer required dialysis and was eventually discharged home after completing a prolonged course of intravenous anti-staphylococcal antibiotics at a rehabilitation facility. Follow-up urine testing on two occasions revealed 1.6 and 1.4 g of protein in 24-hour collections, but serum creatinine remained normal, and microscopy demonstrated no dysmorphic red cells or red-cell casts. Other than transient arthralgia and malar rash, her lupus has been quiescent, and her prednisone dose was tapered to 5 mg daily. Six months after discharge, she returned to school.

COMMENTARY

Using the American College of Rheumatology (ACR) definition, SLE is diagnosed when at least four criteria are met with a sensitivity and specificity above 95%. These criteria were developed for study purposes to differentiate SLE from other rheumatic diseases. At disease onset, a patient may not meet the ACR threshold, but delaying treatment may be harmful. Data conflict on the probability of such patients eventually being classified as having SLE, with estimates ranging from less than 10% to more than 60%.[1,2] With SLE prominent in the differential diagnosis of a critically ill patient, physicians must consider the three most common causes of death in lupus patients: lupus crisis, severe infection, and thrombosis.[3]

Most exacerbations of SLE occur in one system, most commonly the musculoskeletal system, and are mild. However, every year, 10% of patients will require high-dose corticosteroids or cytotoxic agents for severe flares that can occur in any system affected by lupus and 15% of cases may involve multiple sites simultaneously.[4,5] Diagnosing lupus flares remains challenging. Although pulmonary hemorrhage and red blood cell casts may strongly implicate active lupus in the lungs or kidneys, specific clinical and laboratory markers of lupus crisis are lacking. Several global indices reliably measure current disease status but are cumbersome, cannot be relied on solely for treatment decisions, and have not been well studied in hospitalized patients.[6–8] Fever, once a dependable harbinger of active lupus,[9] cannot reliably discriminate lupus flares from infection. In two studies, Rovin et al. found that infection accounted for fever in all but one SLE outpatient taking prednisone and that in hospitalized SLE patients, failure of fevers to resolve within 48 hours of administering 20–40 mg of prednisone daily strongly suggested infection.[10] The laboratory findings provided general support for there being an SLE flare or an infection, but, as the discussant pointed out, these cannot be relied on exclusively to discriminate between the two. Results that suggest infection in an SLE patient include leukocytosis, increased band forms or metamyelocytes, and possibly elevated C-reactive protein. Findings favoring SLE flare include leukopenia, low C3 or C4 (particularly for nephritis or hematologic flares), and elevated anti-double-stranded DNA antibodies for nephritis.[11–13] Without a gold standard for definitively determining a lupus crisis, it is diagnosed when clinical manifestations fit a pattern seen in SLE (nephritis, cerebritis, serositis, vasculitis, pneumonitis), the results of serology studies support this conclusion, and other plausible diagnoses are excluded.

Infection and active disease account for most ICU admissions of lupus patients. SLE and infection intertwine in three ways. First, SLE patients are predisposed to infection, possibly because of a variety of identified genetic abnormalities of immune function.[14] Although community-acquired bacteria and viruses account for most infections, lupus patients are vulnerable to a wide array of atypical and opportunistic pathogens. Clinical factors that augment this intrinsic risk include severity of the underlying SLE, flares of the central nervous system or kidneys, and use of immunosuppressive agents.[14] The use of immunosuppressive agents deserves particular attention, as a recent study found more than 90% of SLE patients admitted to an ICU with severe infection were taking corticosteroids prior to hospitalization.[15] Second, infection may trigger a lupus flare. Third, features of severe lupus flares and infection may overlap. Differentiating between the two may be difficult, and the stakes are high, as SLE patients admitted to ICUs have a risk of death that is substantially higher (47%) than that of those without SLE (29%) and much greater than the overall risk of death for those with SLE, for whom 10-year survival exceeds 90%.[15]

In addition to lupus crisis and infection, the differential diagnosis of acute multisystem disease in a patient with SLE includes catastrophic antiphospholipid syndrome (APS) and thrombotic thrombocytopenic purpura, two thrombotic microangiopathies to which SLE patients are predisposed. Thrombocytopenia and hemolytic anemia with schistocytes should raise suspicion of these diagnoses. Additional findings for TTP include fevers, altered mental status, acute renal failure, and elevated serum lactate dehydrogenase; however, prothrombin time should not be prolonged. Lupus anticoagulant or anticardiolipin antibodies are found in up to 30% of lupus patients, of whom 50%–70% develop APS within 20 years, characterized by thrombosis or spontaneous abortions in the presence of antiphospholipid antibodies.[16] Catastrophic APS is a rare subset of APS involving thromboses of multiple organs simultaneously and has a mortality rate of 50%.

In the present patient, an elevated INR, bleeding, hypotension, and the absence of antiphospholipid antibodies argued against TTP and APS, leading the discussant to focus on SLE and sepsis. Arthralgia, cytopenia, and the results of serology studies suggested a lupus crisis, but hypothermia, hypotension, and DIC pointed to severe infection. Empiric treatment of both conditions with corticosteroids and broad-spectrum antibiotics was

TABLE 9.1 Criteria for Toxic Shock Syndrome[19]

1. Fever >38.9°C
2. Hypotension (SBP < 90 mm Hg)
3. Diffuse erythroderma
4. Desquamation, particularly of palms and soles (occurring 1-2 weeks after onset of illness)
5. Involvement of three or more systems:
   - GI (vomiting or diarrhea at onset)
   - Muscular (CK > twice the upper limit of normal or severe myalgia)
   - Mucus membranes (vaginal, oropharyngeal, or conjunctival hyperemia)
   - Renal (pyuria; BUN or creatinine > twice the upper limit of normal)
   - Hepatic (bilirubin or transaminases > twice the upper limit of normal)
   - Hematologic (platelets < 100,000/mm^3)
   - Central nervous system (altered mental status without localizing deficits unexplained by hypotension or fever)

In addition, negative cultures of blood, throat, and cerebrospinal fluid are expected (except for blood cultures in *S. aureus* TSS, which may be positive).

indicated, and ultimately, the patient's condition was found to meet criteria for TSS and SLE. TSS has rarely been reported in SLE[17,18] and poses a particularly difficult diagnostic challenge because a severe lupus flare can meet the diagnostic criteria for TSS (Table 9.1), especially early on, before the characteristic desquamating rash appears. Afraid to not treat a potentially life-threatening condition, the clinicians initiated empiric treatment toward both severe lupus and sepsis. Attention then shifted to fraying, or unraveling, the knot linking infection and lupus. Ultimately, diagnoses of both TSS and SLE were established.

Key Points

1. The three most common causes of mortality in SLE are lupus crisis, infection, and thrombosis.
2. Lupus flares are easily confused with infection and other causes of acute multisystem disease.
3. In critically ill lupus patients, initial treatment may need to be empirically directed at multiple causes until the diagnosis is clear.

Acknowledgment

The authors thank Michael Chan, MD, and Shelley Gordon, MD, for their input in the manuscript.

REFERENCES

1. Greer JM, Panush RS. Incomplete lupus erythematosus. *Arch Intern Med*. 1989;149:2473–2476.
2. Lom-Orta H, Alarcon-Segovia D, Diaz-Jouanen E. Systemic lupus erythematosus. Differences between patients who do, and who do not, fulfill classification criteria at the time of diagnosis. *J Rheumatol*. 1980;7:831–837.
3. Cervera R, Khamashta MA, Font J, et al. Morbidity and mortality in systemic lupus erythematosus during a 10-year period: A comparison of early and late manifestations in a cohort of 1,000 patients. *Medicine (Baltimore)*. 2003;82:299–308.

4. Gordon C, Sutcliffe N, Skan J, Stoll T, Isenberg DA. Definition and treatment of lupus flares measured by the BILAG index. *Rheumatology*. 2003;42:1372–1379.
5. Ehrenstein MR, Conroy SE, Heath J, Latchman DS, Isenberg DA. The occurrence, nature and distributions of flares in a cohort of patients with systemic lupus erythematosus: a rheumatologic view. *Br J Rheumatol*. 1995;34:257–260.
6. Ward MM, Marx AS, Barry NN. Comparison of the validity and sensitivity to change of 5 activity indices in systemic lupus erythematosus. *J Rheumatol*. 2000;27:664–670.
7. Walz-LeBlanc BA, Gladman DD, Urowitz, MB. Serologically active clinically quiescent systemic lupus erythematosus—predictors of clinical flares. *J Rheumatol*. 1994;21:2239–2241.
8. Esdaile JM, Abrahamowicz M, Joseph L, MacKenzie T, Li Y, Danoff D. Laboratory tests as predictors of disease exacerbations in systemic lupus erythematosus. Why some tests fail. *Arthritis Rheum*. 1996;39:370–378.
9. Stahl NI, Klippel JH, Decker JL. Fever in systemic lupus erythematosus. *Am J Med*. 1979;67:935–940.
10. Rovin BH, Tang Y, Sun J, et al. Clinical significance of fever in the systemic lupus erythematosus patient receiving steroid therapy. *Kidney Int*. 2005;68:747–759.
11. Sidiropoulos PI, Kritikos HD, Boumpas DT. Lupus nephritis flares. *Lupus*. 2005;14:49–52.
12. Ho A, Barr SG, Magder LS, Petri M. A decrease in complement is associated with increased renal and hematologic activity in patients with systemic lupus erythematosus. *Arthritis Rheum*. 2001;44:2350–2357.
13. Petri M, Genovese M, Engle E, Hochberg M. Definition, incidence, and clinical description of flare in systemic lupus erythematosus. A prospective cohort study. *Arthritis Rheum*. 1991;34:937–944.
14. Zandman-Goddard G, Shoenfeld Y. Infections and SLE. *Autoimmunity*. 2005;38:473–485.
15. Hsu CL, Chen KY, Yeh PS, et al. Outcome and prognostic factors in critically ill patients with systemic lupus erythematosus: A retrospective study. *Crit Care*. 2005;9:R177–R183.
16. Levine JS, Branch DW, Rauch J. The antiphospholipid syndrome. *N Engl J Med*. 2002;346:752–763.
17. Chan RMT, Graham HR, Birmingham CL. Toxic shock syndrome in a patient with systemic lupus erythematosus. *Can Med Assoc J*. 1983;129:1201–1202.
18. Huseyin TS, Maynard JP, Leach RD. Toxic shock syndrome in a patient with breast cancer and systemic lupus erythematosus. *Eur J Surg Oncol*. 2001;27:330–331.
19. Case definitions for infectious conditions under public health surveillance. *MMWR Recomm Rep*. 1997;46(RR-10):39.

CHAPTER **10**

BETTER LATE THAN NEVER

ANURADHA RAMASWAMY
Department of Hospital Medicine, Cleveland Clinic, Cleveland, Ohio

MAYTEE BOONYAPREDEE and RAMAKRISHNAN RANGANATH
Department of Internal Medicine, Franklin Square Hospital Center, Baltimore, Maryland

BRIAN J. HARTE
South Pointe Hospital, Cleveland Clinic Health System, Warrensville Heights, Ohio

JAMES C. PILE
Departments of Hospital Medicine and Infectious Diseases, Cleveland Clinic, Cleveland, Ohio

A 59-year-old man presented to the emergency department with the acute onset of right-sided abdominal and flank pain. The pain had begun the previous night, was constant and progressively worsening, and radiated to his right groin. He denied fever, nausea, emesis, or change in his bowel habits, but he did notice mild right lower quadrant discomfort with micturition. Upon further questioning, he also complained of mild dyspnea on climbing stairs and an unspecified recent weight loss.

The most common cause of acute severe right-sided flank and abdominal pain radiating to the groin and associated with dysuria in a middle-aged man is ureteral colic. Other etiologies important to consider include retrocecal appendicitis, pyelonephritis, and, rarely, a dissecting abdominal aortic aneurysm. However, this patient's seemingly recent-onset exertional dyspnea and recent weight loss do not neatly fit any of the above.

His past medical history was significant for diabetes mellitus and pemphigus vulgaris diagnosed 7 months previously. He had been treated with prednisone, and the dose decreased from 100 to 60 mg daily 1 month previously due to poor glycemic control as well as steroid-induced neuropathy and myopathy. His other medications included naproxen sodium and ibuprofen for back pain, azathioprine, insulin, pioglitazone, and glimepiride. He had no past surgical history. He had lived in the United States since his emigration from Thailand in 1971. His last trip to Thailand was 5 years ago. He was a taxi cab driver. He had a 10-pack year history of tobacco use, but had quit 20 years before. He denied history of alcohol or intravenous drug use.

Pemphigus vulgaris is unlikely to be directly related to this patient's presentation, but in light of his poorly controlled diabetes, his azathioprine use, and particularly his high-dose corticosteroids, he is certainly immunocompromised. Accordingly, a disseminated infection, either newly acquired or reactivated, merits consideration. His history of

Clinical Care Conundrums: Challenging Diagnoses in Hospital Medicine, First Edition.
Edited by James C. Pile, Thomas E. Baudendistel, and Brian J. Harte.

residence in, and subsequent travel to, Southeast Asia raises the possibility of several diseases, each of which may be protean in their manifestations; these include tuberculosis, melioidosis, and penicilliosis (infection with *Penicillium marneffei).* The first two may reactivate long after initial exposure, particularly with insults to the immune system. On a slightly less exotic note, domestically acquired infection with histoplasmosis or other endemic fungi is possible.

On examination he was afebrile and had a pulse of 130 beats per minute and a blood pressure of 65/46 mm Hg. His oxygen saturation was 92%. He appeared markedly cushingoid and had mild pallor and generalized weakness. Cardiopulmonary examination was unremarkable. His abdominal exam was notable for distention and hypoactive bowel sounds, with tenderness and firmness to palpation on the right side. Peripheral pulses were normal. Examination of the skin demonstrated ecchymoses over the bilateral forearms and several healed pemphigus lesions on the abdomen and upper extremities.

The patient's severely deranged hemodynamic parameters indicate either current or impending shock, and resuscitative measures should proceed in tandem with diagnostic efforts. The cause of his shock seems most likely to be either hypovolemic (abdominal wall or intra-abdominal hemorrhage, or conceivably massive third spacing from an intra-abdominal catastrophe) or distributive (sepsis or acute adrenal insufficiency if he has missed recent steroid doses). His ecchymoses may simply reflect chronic glucocorticoid use, and also raise suspicion of coagulopathy. Provided the patient can be stabilized to allow this, I would urgently obtain a computed tomography (CT) scan of the abdomen and pelvis.

Initial laboratory studies demonstrated a hemoglobin of 9.1 g/dL; white blood cell count of 8000/μL, with 33% bands, 48% segmented neutrophils, 18% lymphocytes, and 0.7% eosinophils; platelet count of 356,000/μL; sodium of 128 mmol/L; BUN of 52 mg/dL; creatinine of 2.3 mg/dL; and glucose of 232 mg/dL. Coagulation studies were normal, and lactic acid was 1.8 mmol/L (normal range, 0.7–2.1). Fibrinogen was normal at 591 and LDH was 654 (normal range, 313–618 U/L). Total protein and albumin were 3.6 and 1.9 g/dL, respectively. Total bilirubin was 0.6 mg/dL. Random serum cortisol was 20.2 μg/dL. Liver enzymes, amylase, lipase, iron stores, B_{12}, folate, and stool for occult blood were normal. Initial cardiac biomarkers were negative, but subsequent troponin-I was 3.81 ng/mL (elevated, >1.00). Urinalysis showed 0–4 white blood cells per high-powered field.

The laboratory studies provide a variety of useful, albeit nonspecific, information. The high percentage of band forms on white blood cell differential further raises concern for an infectious process, although severe noninfectious stress can also cause this. While we do not know whether the patient's renal failure is acute, I suspect that it is and may result from a variety of insults including sepsis, hypotension, and volume depletion. His moderately elevated troponin-I likely reflects supply–demand mismatch or sepsis. I would like to see an electrocardiogram, and I remain very interested in obtaining abdominal imaging.

Chest radiography showed pulmonary vascular congestion without evidence of pneumothorax. CT scan of the abdomen and pelvis showed retroperitoneal fluid bilaterally (Fig. 10.1). This was described as suspicious for ascites versus hemorrhage, but no obvious source of bleeding was identified. There was also a small amount of right perinephric fluid, but no evidence of a renal mass. The abdominal aorta was normal; there was no lymphadenopathy.

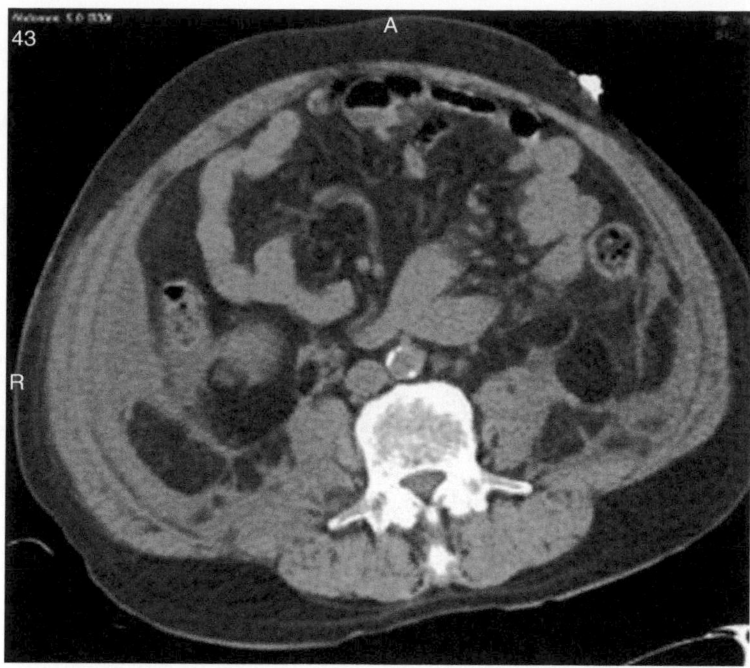

FIGURE 10.1 Computed tomography (CT) scan of the abdomen and pelvis shows bilateral retroperitoneal fluid collections, right greater than left.

The CT image appears to speak against simple ascites, and seems most consistent with either blood or an infectious process. Consequently, the loculated right retroperitoneal collection should be aspirated, and fluid sent for fungal, acid-fast, and modified acid-fast (i.e., for *Nocardia*) stains and culture, in addition to Gram stain and routine aerobic and anaerobic cultures.

The patient was admitted to the intensive care unit. Stress-dose steroids were administered, and he improved after resuscitation with fluid and blood. His renal function normalized. Urine and blood cultures returned negative. His hematocrit and multiple repeat CT scans of the abdomen remained stable. A retroperitoneal hemorrhage was diagnosed, and surgical intervention was deemed unnecessary. Both adenosine thallium stress test and echocardiogram were normal. He was continued on 60-mg prednisone daily and discharged home with outpatient follow-up.

This degree of improvement with volume expansion (and steroids) suggests that the patient was markedly volume depleted on presentation. Although a formal adrenocorticotropic hormone (ACTH) stimulation test was apparently not performed, the random cortisol level suggests that adrenal insufficiency was unlikely to have been primarily responsible. While retroperitoneal hemorrhage is possible, the loculated appearance of the collection suggests that infection is more likely.

Three weeks later, he was readmitted with recurrent right-sided abdominal and flank pain. His temperature was 101.3°F, and he was tachycardic and hypotensive. His examination was similar to that at the time of his previous presentation. Laboratory data revealed white blood cell count of 13,100/μL with 43% bands, hemoglobin of 9.2 g/dL, glucose of 343 mg/dL, bicarbonate of 25 mmol/L, normal anion gap and renal function, and lactic acid of 4.5 mmol/L. Liver function tests

were normal except for an albumin of 3.0 g/dL. CT scan of the abdomen revealed loculated retroperitoneal fluid collections, increased in size since the prior scan.

The patient is once again evidencing at least early shock, manifested in his deranged hemodynamics and elevated lactate level. I remain puzzled by the fact that he appeared to respond to fluids alone at the time of his initial hospital stay, unless adrenal insufficiency played a greater role than I suspected. Of note, acute adrenal insufficiency could explain much of the current picture, including fever. Also bland (uninfected) hematomas are an underappreciated cause of both fever and leukocytosis. Having said this, I remain concerned that his retroperitoneal fluid collections represent abscesses. The most accessible of these should be sampled.

Aspiration of the retroperitoneal fluid yielded purulent material that grew *Klebsiella pneumoniae*. The cultures were negative for mycobacteria and fungus. Blood and urine cultures were negative. Drains were placed, and he was followed as an outpatient. His fever and leukocytosis subsided, and he completed a 6-week course of trimethoprim-sulfamethoxazole. CT imaging confirmed complete evacuation of the fluid.

Retroperitoneal abscesses frequently present in smoldering fashion, although patients may be quite ill by the time of presentation. Most of these are secondary, that is, they arise from another abnormality in the retroperitoneum. Most commonly, this occurs in the large bowel, kidney, pancreas, or spine. I would carefully scour his follow-up imaging for additional clues and if unrevealing, proceed to colonoscopy.

He returned 1 month after drain removal, with 2–3 days of nausea and abdominal pain. His abdomen was moderately distended but nontender, and multiple persistent petechial and purpuric lesions were present on the upper back, chest, torso, and arms. Abdominal CT scan revealed small bowel obstruction and a collection of fluid in the left paracolic gutter extending into the left retrorenal space.

The patient does not appear to have obvious risk factors for developing a small bowel obstruction. No mention is made of the presence or absence of a transition point on the CT scan, and this should be ascertained. His left-sided abdominal fluid collection is probably infectious in nature, and I continue to be suspicious of a large bowel (or distal small bowel) source, via either gut perforation or bacterial translocation. The collection needs to be percutaneously drained for both diagnostic and therapeutic reasons, and broadly cultured. Finally, we need to account for the described dermatologic manifestations. The purpuric/petechial lesions sound vasculitic rather than thrombocytopenic in origin based on location; conversely, they may simply reflect a corticosteroid-related adverse effect. I would like to know whether the purpura was palpable and to repeat a complete blood count with peripheral smear.

Laboratory data showed hemoglobin of 9.3 g/dL, a platelet count of 444,000/μL, and normal coagulation studies. The purpura was nonpalpable (Fig. 10.2). The patient had a nasogastric tube placed for decompression, with bilious drainage. His left retroperitoneal fluid was drained, with cultures yielding *Enterococcus faecalis* and *Enterobacter cloacae*. The patient was treated with a course of broad-spectrum antibiotics. His obstruction improved and the retroperitoneal collection resolved on follow-up imaging. However, 2 days later, he had recurrent pain; abdominal CT showed a recurrence of small bowel obstruction with an unequivocal transition point in the distal jejunum. A small fluid collection was noted in the left retroperitoneum with a trace of gas in it. He improved

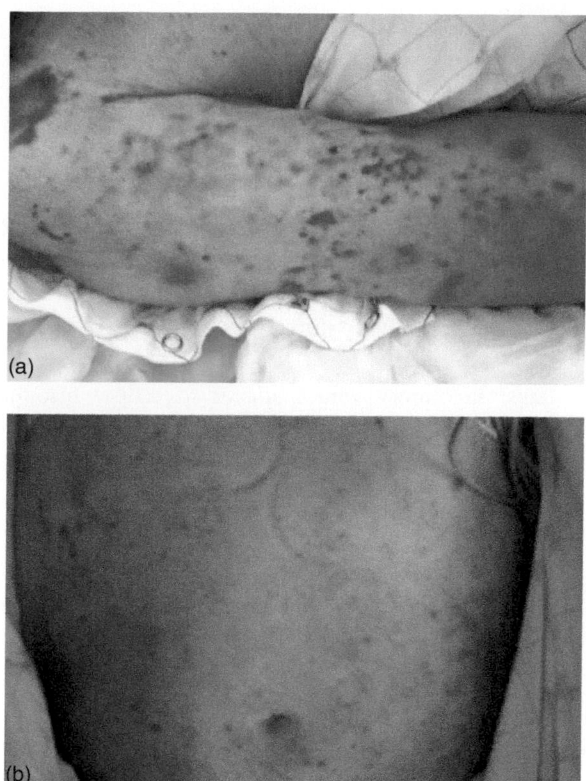

FIGURE 10.2 Multiple petechial and purpuric lesions in skin of (a) right upper extremity and shoulder and (b) abdomen.

with nasogastric suction, his prednisone was tapered to 30 mg daily, and he was discharged home.

The isolation of both *Enterococcus* and *Enterobacter* species from his fluid collection, along with the previous isolation of *Klebsiella*, strongly suggest a bowel source for his recurrent abscesses. Based on this CT report, the patient has clear evidence of at least partial small bowel obstruction. He lacks a history of prior abdominal surgery or other more typical reasons for obstruction caused by extrinsic compression, such as hernia, although it is possible his recurrent abdominal infections may have led to obstruction due to scarring and adhesions. An intraluminal cause of obstruction also needs to be considered, with causes including malignancy (lymphoma, carcinoid, and adenocarcinoma), Crohn's disease, and infections including tuberculosis, as well as parasites such as *Taenia* and *Strongyloides*. While the purpura is concerning, given the nonpalpable character along with a normal platelet count and coagulation studies, I will provisionally attribute it to high-dose corticosteroid use.

He was admitted a fourth time a week after being discharged, with nausea, generalized weakness, and weight loss. At presentation, he had a blood pressure of 95/65 mm Hg. His white blood cell count was 5900/μL, with 79% neutrophils and 20% bands. An AM cortisol was 18.8 μ/dL. He was thought to have adrenal insufficiency from steroid withdrawal, was treated with intravenous fluids and steroids, and discharged on a higher dose of prednisone at 60 mg daily. One week later, he again returned to the hospital with watery diarrhea, emesis, and generalized

weakness. His blood pressure was 82/50 mm Hg, and his abdomen appeared benign. He also had an erythematous rash over his mid-abdomen. Laboratory data was significant for a sodium of 127 mmol/L, potassium of 3.0 mmol/L, chloride of 98 mmol/L, bicarbonate of 26 mmol/L, glucose of 40 mg/dL, lactate of 14 mmol/L, and albumin of 1.0 g/dL. Stool assay for *Clostridium difficile* was negative. A CT scan of the abdomen and pelvis showed small bilateral pleural effusions and small bowel fluid consistent with gastroenteritis, but without signs of obstruction. Esophagogastroduodenoscopy (EGD) showed bile backwash into the stomach, as well as inflammatory changes in the proximal and mid-stomach, and inflammatory reaction and edema in the proximal duodenum. Colonoscopy showed normal appearing ileum and colon.

The patient's latest laboratory values appear to reflect his chronic illness and superimposed diarrhea. I am perplexed by his markedly elevated serum lactate value in association with a normal bicarbonate and low anion gap and would repeat the lactate level to ensure this is not spurious. His hypoglycemia probably reflects a failure to adjust or discontinue his diabetic medications, although both hypoglycemia and type B lactic acidosis are occasionally manifestations of a paraneoplastic syndrome. The normal colonoscopic findings are helpful in exonerating the colon, provided the preparation was adequate. Presumably, the abnormal areas of the stomach and duodenum were biopsied; I remain suspicious that the answer may lie in the jejunum.

The patient was treated with intravenous fluids and stress-dose steroids, and electrolyte abnormalities were corrected. Biopsies from the EGD and colonoscopy demonstrated numerous larvae within the mucosa of the body and antrum of the stomach, as well as duodenum. There were also rare detached larvae seen in the esophagus, and a few larvae within the ileal mucosa.

The patient appears to have *Strongyloides* hyperinfection, something he is at clear risk for, given his country of origin and his high-dose corticosteroids. In retrospect, I was dissuaded from seriously considering a diagnosis of parasitic infection in large part because of the absence of peripheral eosinophilia, but this may not be seen in cases of hyperinfection. Additional clues, again in retrospect, were the repeated abscesses with bowel flora and the seemingly nonspecific abdominal rash. I would treat with a course of ivermectin and carefully monitor his response.

The characteristics of the larvae were suggestive of *Strongyloides* species (Fig. 10.3). A subsequent stool test for ova and parasites was positive for *Strongyloides* larvae. The patient was given a single dose of ivermectin. An endocrinology consultant felt that he did not have adrenal insufficiency, and it was recommended that his steroids be tapered off. He was discharged home once he clinically improved.

Although one or two doses of ivermectin typically suffice for uncomplicated strongyloidiasis, the risk of failure in hyperinfection mandates a longer treatment course. I do not believe that this patient has been adequately treated, although the removal of his steroids will be helpful.

He was readmitted 3 days later with recrudescent symptoms, and his stool remained positive for *Strongyloides.* He received 2 weeks of ivermectin and albendazole and was ultimately discharged to a rehabilitation facility after a complicated hospital stay. Nine months later, the patient was reported to be doing well.

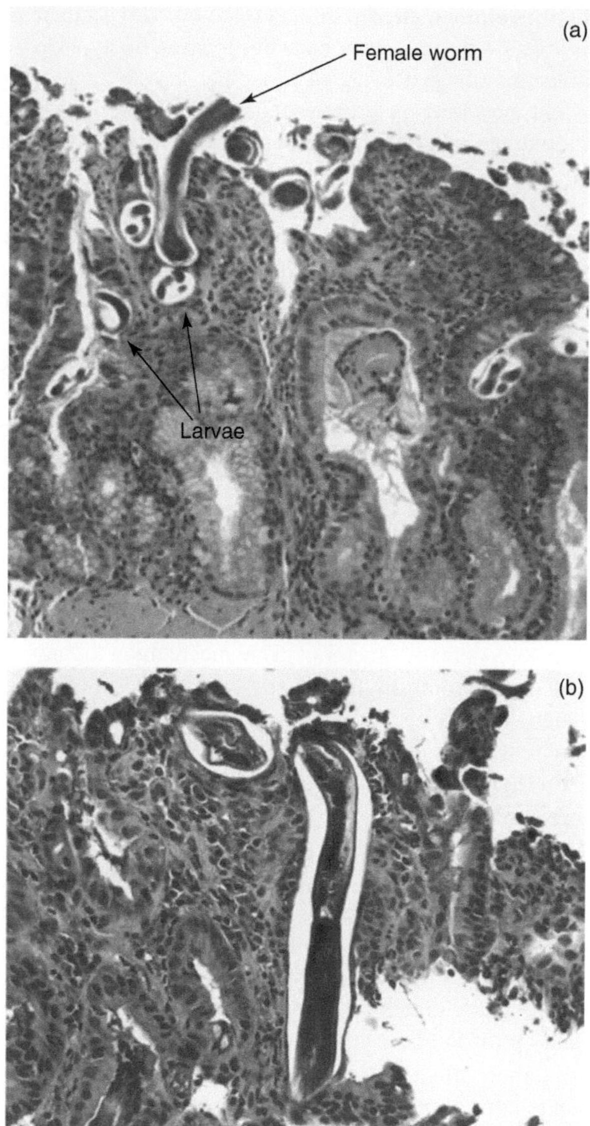

FIGURE 10.3 (a) Examination of duodenal biopsy shows several larvae and adult *Strongyloides* worms. Only adult females are parasitic and responsible for host infection, while adult male worms are generally found free-living in the soil. (b) Magnified view of duodenal biopsy shows inflammatory infiltrates in lamina propria and adult worms burrowed in the mucosa.

COMMENTARY

This patient's immigration status from the developing world, high-dose corticosteroid use, and complex clinical course all suggested the possibility of an underlying chronic infectious process. Although the discussant recognized this early on and later briefly mentioned strongyloidiasis as a potential cause of intestinal obstruction, the diagnosis of *Strongyloides* hyperinfection was not suspected until incontrovertible evidence for it was obtained on EGD. Failure to make the diagnosis earlier by both the involved clinicians and the discussant probably stemmed largely from two factors: the absence of eosinophilia and the lack of recognition that purpura may be seen in cases of hyperinfection, presumably reflecting larval infiltration of the dermis.[1] Although eosinophilia accompanies most cases of strongyloidiasis and may be very pronounced, patients with hyperinfection syndrome frequently fail to mount an eosinophilic response due to underlying immunosuppression, with eosinophilia absent in 70% of such patients in a study from Taiwan.[2]

Strongyloides stercoralis is an intestinal nematode that causes strongyloidiasis. It affects as many as 100 million people globally,[3] mainly in tropical and subtropical areas, but it is also endemic in the Southeastern United States, Europe, and Japan. In nonendemic regions, it more commonly affects travelers, immigrants, or military personnel.[4,5]

The life cycle of *S. stercoralis* is complex. Infective larvae penetrate the skin through contact with contaminated soil, enter the venous system via lymphatics, and travel to the lung,[4,6] where they ascend the tracheobronchial tree and migrate to the gut. In the intestine, larvae develop into adult female worms that burrow into the intestinal mucosa. These worms lay eggs that develop into noninfective rhabditiform larvae, which are then expelled in the stool. Some of the rhabditiform larvae, however, develop into infective filariform larvae, which may penetrate colonic mucosa or perianal skin, enter the bloodstream, and lead to the cycle of autoinfection and chronic strongyloidiasis (carrier state). Autoinfection typically involves a low parasite burden and is controlled by both host immune factors and parasitic factors.[7] The mechanism of autoinfection can lead to the persistence of strongyloidiasis for decades after the initial infection, as has been documented in former World War II prisoners.[8]

Factors leading to the impairment of cell-mediated immunity predispose chronically infected individuals to hyperinfection, as occurred in this patient. The most important of these are corticosteroid administration and human T-lymphotropic virus type 1 (HTLV-1) infection, both of which cause significant derangement in TH1/TH2 immune system balance.[5,9] In the hyperinfection syndrome, the burden of parasites increases dramatically, leading to a variety of clinical manifestations. Gastrointestinal phenomena frequently predominate, including watery diarrhea, anorexia, weight loss, nausea/vomiting, gastrointestinal bleeding, and occasionally small bowel obstruction. Pulmonary manifestations are likewise common and include cough, dyspnea, and wheezing. Cutaneous findings are not uncommon, classically pruritic linear lesions of the abdomen, buttocks, and lower extremities, which may be rapidly migratory ("larva currens"), although purpura and petechiae as displayed by our patient appear to be underrecognized findings in hyperinfection.[2,5] Gram-negative bacillary meningitis has been well reported as a complication of migrating larvae, and a wide variety of other organs may rarely be involved.[5,10]

The presence of chronic strongyloidiasis should be suspected in patients with ongoing gastrointestinal and/or pulmonary symptoms, or unexplained eosinophilia with a potential exposure history, such as immigrants from Southeast Asia. Diagnosis in these individuals is currently most often made serologically, although stool exam provides a somewhat higher specificity for active infection, at the expense of lower sensitivity.[3,11] In the setting of hyperinfection, stool studies are almost uniformly positive for *S. stercoralis*, and sputum may be diagnostic as well. Consequently, failure to reach the diagnosis usually reflects a lack of clinical suspicion.[5]

Currently, the therapy of choice for strongyloidiasis is ivermectin. A single dose repeated once, 2 weeks later, is highly efficacious in eradicating chronic infection. Treatment of hyperinfection is more challenging and less well studied, but clearly necessitates a more prolonged course of treatment. Many experts advocate treating until worms are no longer present in the stool; some have suggested the combination of ivermectin and albendazole as this patient received, although this has not been examined in a controlled manner.

The diagnosis of *Strongyloides* hyperinfection is typically delayed or missed because of the failure to consider it, with reported mortality rates as high as 50% in hyperinfection and 87% in disseminated disease.[3,12,13] This patient fortunately was diagnosed, albeit in delayed fashion, proving the maxim "better late than never." His case highlights the need for increased clinical awareness of strongyloidiasis and specifically the need to consider the possibility of chronic *Strongyloides* infection prior to administering immunosuppressive medications. In particular, serologic screening of individuals from highly endemic areas for strongyloidiasis, when initiating extended courses of corticosteroids, is prudent.[13]

Key Points

1. Chronic strongyloidiasis is common in the developing world (particularly, Southeast Asia) and places infected individuals at significant risk of life-threatening hyperinfection if not recognized and treated prior to the initiation of immunosuppressive medication, especially corticosteroids.
2. *Strongyloides* hyperinfection syndrome may be protean in its manifestations, and hypereosinophilia is often absent, but gastrointestinal, pulmonary, and cutaneous signs and symptoms are most common.
3. Diagnosis of strongyloidiasis is most often confirmed serologically, whereas the hyperinfection syndrome can be diagnosed reliably with stool studies.

REFERENCES

1. Galimberti R, Ponton A, Zaputovich FA, et al. Disseminated strongyloidiasis in immunocompromised patients—report of three cases. *Int J Dermatol*. 2009;48(9):975–978.
2. Tsai HC, Lee SS, Liu YC, et al. Clinical manifestations of strongyloidiasis in southern Taiwan. *J Microbiol Immunol Infect*. 2002;35(1):29–36.
3. Siddiqui AA, Berk SL. Diagnosis of Strongyloides stercoralis infection. *Clin Infect Dis*. 2001;33(7): 1040–1047.
4. Vadlamudi RS, Chi DS, Krishnaswamy G. Intestinal strongyloidiasis and hyperinfection syndrome. *Clin Mol Allergy*. 2006;4:8.
5. Keiser PB, Nutman TB. Strongyloides stercoralis in the immunocom-promised population. *Clin Microbiol Rev*. 2004;17(1):208–217.
6. Concha R, Harrington W Jr., Rogers AI. Intestinal strongyloidiasis: Recognition, management and determinants of outcome. *J Clin Gastroenterol*. 2005;39(3):203–211.
7. Genta RM. Dysregulation of strongyloidiasis: A new hypothesis. *Clin Microbiol Rev*. 1992;5(4):345–355.
8. Robson D, Welch E, Beeching NJ, Gill GV. Consequences of captivity: Health effects of Far East imprisonment in World War II. *Q J Med*. 2009;102:87–96.
9. Marcos LA, Terashima A, Dupont HL, Gotuzzo E. Strongyloides hyperinfection syndrome: An emerging global infectious disease. *Trans R Soc Trop Med Hyg*. 2008;102(4):314–318.
10. Newberry AM, Williams DN, Stauffer WM, Boulware DR, Hendel-Paterson BR, Walker PF. Strongyloides hyperinfection presenting as acute respiratory failure and Gram-negative sepsis. *Chest*. 2005;128(5):3681–3684.
11. van Doorn HR, Koelewijn R, Hofwegen H, et al. Use of enzyme-linked immunosorbent assay and dipstick assay for detection of *Strongyloides stercoralis* infection in humans. *J Clin Microbiol*. 2007;45:438–442.
12. Lim S, Katz K, Krajden S, Fuksa M, Keystone J, Kain K. Complicated and fatal *Strongyloides* infection in Canadians: Risk factors, diagnosis and management. *Can Med Assoc J*. 2004;171:479–484.
13. Boulware DR, Stauffer WM, Hendel-Paterson BR, et al. Maltreatment of *Strongyloides* infection: Case series and worldwide physicians-in-training survey. *Am J Med*. 2007;120(6):545.e1–545.e8.

CHAPTER **11**

THINKING INSIDE THE BOX

DAMON M. KWAN
Division of Cardiology, Kaiser Permanente Medical Center, Los Angeles, California; Department of Medicine, California Pacific Medical Center, San Francisco, California

GURPREET DHALIWAL
Department of Medicine, University of California, San Francisco, California; San Francisco VA Medical Center, San Francisco, California

THOMAS E. BAUDENDISTEL
Department of Medicine, Kaiser Permanente Medical Center, Oakland, California

A 65-year-old man was referred for evaluation of worsening ascites and end-stage liver disease. The patient had been well until 1 year ago, when he developed lower extremity edema and abdominal distention. After evaluation by his primary care physician, he was given a diagnosis of cryptogenic cirrhosis. He underwent several paracenteses and was placed on furosemide and spironolactone. The patient had been stable on his diuretic regimen until 2 weeks previously, when he suddenly developed worsening edema and ascites, along with dizziness, nausea, and hypotension. His physician stopped the diuretics and referred him to the hospital.

Before diagnosing a patient with cryptogenic cirrhosis, it is necessary to exclude common etiologies of cirrhosis such as alcohol, viral hepatitis, and nonalcoholic fatty liver disease and numerous uncommon causes, including Wilson's disease, hemochromatosis, Budd–Chiari syndrome, and biliary cirrhosis. It is also important to remember that patients with liver disease are not immune to extrahepatic causes of ascites, such as peritoneal carcinomatosis and tuberculous ascites. Simultaneously, reasons for chronic liver disease decompensating acutely must be considered: medication nonadherence, excess salt intake, hepatotoxicity from acetaminophen or alcohol, and other acute insults, such as hepatocellular carcinoma, an intervening infection (especially spontaneous bacterial peritonitis), ascending cholangitis, or a flare of chronic viral hepatitis.

Past medical and surgical history included diabetes mellitus (diagnosed 10 years previously), obstructive sleep apnea, hypertension, hypothyroidism, and mild chronic kidney disease. Medications included levothyroxine, lactulose, sulfamethoxazole, pioglitazone (started 4 months prior), and ibuprofen. Furosemide and spironolactone had been discontinued 2 weeks previously. He currently resided in the Central Valley of California. He had lived in Thailand from age 7 to 17 years and traveled to India more than 1 year ago. He did not smoke and had never

Clinical Care Conundrums: Challenging Diagnoses in Hospital Medicine, First Edition.
Edited by James C. Pile, Thomas E. Baudendistel, and Brian J. Harte.

used intravenous drugs or received a blood transfusion. He rarely drank alcohol. He worked as a chemist. There was no family history of liver disease.

There is no obvious explanation for the underlying liver disease or the acute decompensation. Sulfamethoxazole is a rare cause of allergic or granulomatous hepatitis. Pioglitazone is a thiazolinedione that in earlier formulations was linked to hepatitis but can be excluded as a cause of this patient's cirrhosis because it was started after liver disease was detected. As a chemist, he might have been exposed to carbon tetrachloride, a known hepatotoxin. Obstructive sleep apnea causes pulmonary hypertension, but severe ascites and acute hepatic decompensation would be unusual. Ibuprofen might precipitate worsening renal function and fluid accumulation. Time in Thailand and India raises the possibility of tuberculous ascites.

The patient had no headache, vision changes, abdominal pain, emesis, melena, hematochezia, chest pain, palpitations, dysuria, polyuria, pruritus, dark urine, or rashes. He reported difficulty with concentration when lactulose was decreased. He noted worsening exercise tolerance with dyspnea after 10 steps and reported a weight gain of 12 pounds in the past 2 weeks.

On examination, temperature was 36.8°C; blood pressure, 129/87 mm Hg; heart rate, 85 beats per minute; respirations, 20 per minute; and oxygen saturation, 94% on room air. He was uncomfortable but alert. There was no scleral icterus or conjunctival pallor. Jugular venous pressure was elevated. The lungs were clear, and the heart was regular, with no murmur, rub, or gallops. The abdomen was massively distended with a fluid wave; the liver and spleen could not be palpated. There was pitting edema of the sacrum and lower extremities. There was no asterixis, palmar erythema, spider angiomata, or skin discoloration.

The additional history and physical exam suggest that the primary problem may lie outside the liver, especially as signs of advanced liver disease (other than ascites) are absent. Dyspnea on exertion is consistent with the physical stress of a large volume of ascites or could be secondary to several pulmonary complications associated with liver disease, including portopulmonary hypertension, hepatopulmonary syndrome, or hepatic hydrothorax. Alternatively, the dyspnea raises the possibility that the ascites is not related to a primary liver disorder but rather to anemia or to a cardiac disorder, such as chronic left ventricular failure, isolated right-sided heart failure, or constrictive pericarditis. These diagnoses are suggested by the elevated jugular venous pressure, which is atypical of cirrhosis.

Although portal hypertension accounts for most cases of ascites, peritoneal fluid should be examined to exclude peritoneal carcinomatosis and tuberculous ascites. I am interested in the results of an echocardiogram.

Initial laboratory studies demonstrated that the sodium concentration was 136 mEq/dL; potassium, 4.7 mEq/dL; chloride, 99 mEq/dL; bicarbonate, 24 mEq/dL; blood urea nitrogen, 54 mg/dL; creatinine, 3.3 mg/dL (increased from baseline of 1.6 mg/dL 4 months previously); white cell count, 7000/mm^3; hemoglobin, 10.5 g/dL; MCV, 89 fL; platelet count, 205,000/mm^3; bilirubin, 0.6 mg/dL; aspartate aminotransferase, 15 U/L; alanine aminotransferase, 8 U/L; alkaline phosphatase, 102 U/L; albumin, 4.2 g/dL; total protein, 8.2 g/dL; international normalized ratio, 1.2; and partial thromboplastin time, 31.8 seconds. A urine dipstick demonstrated 1+ protein. The chest radiograph was normal. Electrocardiogram (ECG) had borderline low voltage with nonspecific T-wave abnormalities. Additional studies showed a serum iron concentration of 49 mg/dL, transferrin saturation of 16%, total iron binding capacity of 310 mg/dL, and ferritin of 247 mg/mL. Hemoglobin

A1c was 7.0%. Acute and chronic antibodies to hepatitis A, B, and C viruses were negative. The following study results were normal or negative: antinuclear antibody, alpha-1-antitrypsin, ceruloplasmin, alpha-fetoprotein, carcinoembryonic antigen, and 24-hour urinary copper. The thyroid function studies were normal. A purified protein derivative (PPD) skin test was nonreactive.

There continues to be a paucity of evidence of a primary liver disorder. The hepatic enzymes and tests of liver synthetic function are normal, and there is no pancytopenia, as might result from hypersplenism. I remain most suspicious of either a primary cardiac or pericardial disorder with secondary hepatic congestion or a disease that simultaneously affects the heart and liver.

The reasons for the low voltage on the ECG include processes that infiltrate the myocardium (amyloidosis, sarcoidosis, hemochromatosis, and myxedema fluid) and processes that increase the distance between the myocardium and surface electrodes, such as adipose tissue, air (from emphysema or pneumothorax), or pericardial effusion. Pericardial effusion may present subacutely with predominant features of right ventricular failure. Low voltage, liver disease, and possible heart failure raise the possibility of amyloidosis or hemochromatosis. The low transferrin saturation renders hemochromatosis unlikely. Although normal alkaline phosphatase and serum albumin are not characteristic when AL amyloid affects the liver and kidneys, serum and urine protein electrophoresis and immunofixation should be considered.

With paracentesis, 3.5 L of ascitic fluid was removed. The red cell count was 4000/mm^3, and white blood cell count was 505/mm^3, of which 25% were polymorphonuclear cells, 22% were lymphocytes, and 53% were monocytes. Additional peritoneal fluid chemistries included albumin of 3.0 g/dL and total protein of 5.3 g/dL. Abdominal Doppler ultrasound demonstrated a liver of normal size and echogenicity with patent hepatic arteries, hepatic veins, and portal vein. There was mild splenomegaly with normal kidneys. Evaluation for a possible liver transplant was initiated. Blood, urine, and peritoneal fluid cultures demonstrated no growth. Echocardiography demonstrated borderline concentric left ventricular hypertrophy, normal right and left ventricular function, dilated superior and inferior vena cavae, and no pericardial effusion or thickening.

The serum-ascites albumin gradient (SAAG) of 1.2 is consistent with portal hypertension as the cause of the ascites. The Doppler findings exclude postsinusoidal causes of portal hypertension from hepatic vein obstruction or thrombosis. The combination of the elevated SAAG, elevated jugular venous pressure, borderline low voltage on ECG, and elevated peritoneal total protein make cardiac and pericardial diseases the leading considerations. Given the normal ventricular function, I am concerned about elevated intracardiac pressures resulting from pericardial disease or restrictive cardiomyopathy. At this point, right heart catheterization would be useful for assessing intracardiac pressures.

On the fourth hospital day, paracentesis was repeated and 15 L of fluid was removed. A transjugular liver biopsy demonstrated diffuse patchy fibrosis consistent with early cirrhosis and minor intralobular changes with minimal ballooning. There was no steatosis, active inflammation, granulomata, iron deposition, or evidence of viral hepatitis. Right heart catheterization revealed a right atrial pressure of 18 cm H_20, right ventricular pressure of 34/20 cm H_20, pulmonary artery pressure of 34/18 cm H_20 (mean, 25), pulmonary capillary wedge pressure of 20 cm H_20, cardiac output of 5.8 L/min, and cardiac index of 2.5 L/min/m^2.

The mild hepatic histologic abnormalities do not support an intrinsic liver disease as the cause of his massive ascites and end-stage liver disease physiology. Cardiac catheterization demonstrates equalization of diastolic pressures, which suggests constrictive pericarditis or restrictive cardiomyopathy. Despite the normal chest radiograph and non-reactive PPD, tuberculosis would be my leading explanation for constrictive pericarditis, given the time spent in areas endemic with TB. Although lateral chest radiography may demonstrate pericardial calcifications, magnetic resonance imaging (MRI) is the best imaging modality to detect constrictive pericarditis. Alternately, cardiac amyloidosis could cause restrictive cardiomyopathy and has not been definitively excluded. A cardiac MRI to assess the pericardium would be my next test, and I would request Congo red stains of the liver biopsy. If these tests are unrevealing, endomyocardial biopsy may be necessary.

The cardiac MRI revealed a severely thickened 7-mm pericardium (normal, <3 mm) most prominent over the right atrium and ventricle. The right ventricle was described as "bullet-shaped," suggesting constrictive pericardial disease (Fig. 11.1). Left heart catheterization to evaluate coronary anatomy and left ventricular pressures revealed no significant coronary arterial disease and demonstrated an elevated left ventricular end-diastolic pressure consistent with constrictive pericarditis. Endomyocardial biopsy showed no evidence of infiltrative disease, granulomata, or other significant abnormality. The following day, the patient underwent pericardiectomy. Postoperatively, his ascites was easily managed with low doses of diuretics. The pericardial tissue revealed chronic inflammatory cells and dense collagenous fibrosis characteristic of constrictive pericarditis without evidence of malignancy or granulomatous disease. Pericardial cultures were negative for bacteria, viruses, fungi, and mycobacteria.

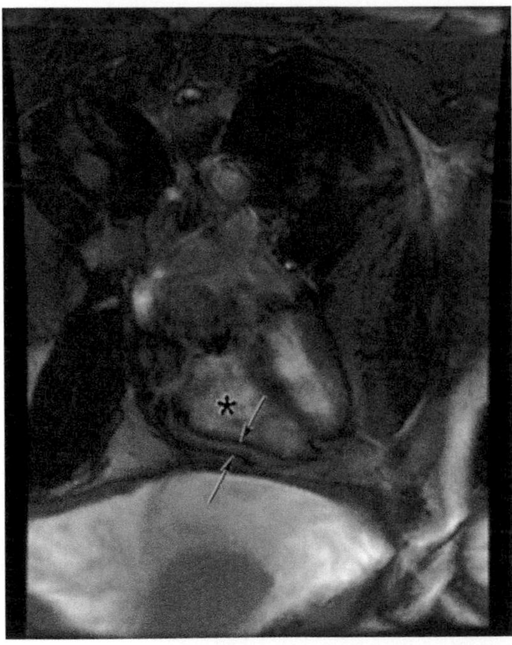

FIGURE 11.1 MRI of the heart. Cardiac MRI demonstrates a thickened pericardium (arrows), measuring 7 mm in its greatest dimension, and a "bullet-shaped" right ventricle (asterisk).

TABLE 11.1 Etiologies of Constrictive Pericarditis in the United States, 1985–2000

- Idiopathic or viral, 46%–50%
- Postcardiac surgery, 18%–37%
- Mediastinal irradiation, 9%–13%
- Connective tissue disorders (most commonly rheumatoid arthritis), 3%–7%
- Infections (tuberculous, bacterial, and fungal), 3%–4%
- Miscellaneous (malignancy, trauma, drug-induced, asbestos)

Data based on 298 patients seen at two surgical referral centers.[1,2]

DISCUSSION

Constrictive pericarditis is characterized by chronic fibrous thickening of the once-elastic pericardial sac and can occur following any disease process that affects the pericardium (Table 11.1).[1,2] The challenge in the diagnosis of constrictive pericarditis lies in the recognition of this slowly progressive and uncommon disease. In many cases, nonspecific symptoms of reduced cardiac output and insidious right-sided heart failure are present for 12 months or longer before a diagnosis is established.[1,3] A typical presentation of constrictive pericarditis is peripheral edema, ascites, and hepatomegaly, a combination that may understandably lead to a misdiagnosis of chronic liver disease and even subject a patient to the unnecessary risk of a liver biopsy, as in this case.

Cryptogenic cirrhosis, the initial diagnosis of this patient, is a term used only after excluding the common and uncommon causes of cirrhosis (Table 11.2).[4–6] With expanded knowledge of the causes of cirrhosis, especially nonalcoholic fatty liver disease, the number of cases of cirrhosis considered to be cryptogenic has decreased from nearly one-third of all cases in 1960 to approximately 5% in a modern series.[7,8] Chronic or repetitive heart failure can lead to progressive hepatic fibrosis and cirrhosis. Distinguishing features compared to other causes of cirrhosis include an ascitic protein concentration

TABLE 11.2 Etiology of Cirrhosis

Most Common

- Alcohol
- Chronic hepatitis B or C
- Nonalcoholic fatty liver disease
- Primary biliary cirrhosis
- Chronic biliary obstruction (eg, primary sclerosing cholangitis)
- Hemochromatosis

Less Common

- Autoimmune hepatitis
- Inherited metabolic disorders (eg, alpha-1-antitrypsin deficiency, Wilson's disease)
- Drugs and toxins (eg, amiodarone, methotrexate)
- Infiltrative disorders (eg, amyloidosis, sarcoidosis)
- Infection (eg, schistosomiasis)
- Vascular abnormalities (eg, veno-occlusive disease, Budd–Chiari syndrome)
- Congestive hepatopathy (cardiac cirrhosis) that is due to right-sided heart failure, severe tricuspid regurgitation, or constrictive pericarditis
- Idiopathic/miscellaneous (eg, polycystic liver disease)

Adapted from references 5–7.

greater than 2.5 g/dL, relatively preserved synthetic function, and infrequent stigmata of end-stage liver disease such as spider angiomata or pronounced jaundice.[9,10]

A key exam feature that distinguishes cardiac cirrhosis from other causes of liver failure is an elevated jugular venous pressure. Hepatic causes of cirrhosis induce increased nitric oxide production, which leads to splanchnic and peripheral arterial vasodilatation with a reduced effective circulating volume and normal or low jugular venous pressure.[11,12] Therefore, a patient with cirrhosis and ascites and an elevated jugular venous pressure should prompt echocardiographic evaluation.[13]

When echocardiography excludes ventricular dysfunction, valvular abnormalities, and pulmonary hypertension, constrictive pericarditis and restrictive cardiomyopathy remain important diagnostic considerations.

In both constrictive pericarditis and restrictive cardiomyopathy, ventricular filling is limited. Pressures in the chambers rise abruptly and rapidly during ventricular filling until equilibrium is reached in early diastole. This can be conceptualized as the cardiac chambers being constrained by the limitations of a rigid external box. In constrictive pericarditis, the rigid external box is the fibrosed and thickened pericardial sac, which loses its elasticity and impairs filling of the ventricles. In restrictive cardiomyopathy, the stiff myocardium limits ventricular filling.

There is considerable overlap in the clinical, echocardiographic, and hemodynamic findings of constrictive pericarditis and restrictive cardiomyopathy.[14] Both may present insidiously with progressive heart failure. Echocardiography demonstrates impaired diastolic function. Cardiac hemodynamics demonstrate abrupt and rapid early diastolic filling, elevated and equal ventricular end-diastolic pressures, and reduced stroke volume and cardiac output. A diagnosis of constrictive pericarditis is favored when a marked inspiratory increase in right ventricular pressures and decrease in left ventricular pressures are seen on heart catheterization or when a similar inspiratory increase in transvalvular flow velocities across the tricuspid valve compared with the mitral valve is shown by echocardiography. This finding results from normal inspiratory increases in intrathoracic pressures, which are unable to be transmitted through the rigid pericardium but continue to augment venous return to the right side of the heart. As many as one-third of patients with pericardial constriction lack these characteristic findings on echocardiogram.[14]

The results of pericardial imaging may suggest a diagnosis of constrictive pericarditis. Lateral chest radiography demonstrates pericardial calcifications in less than 30% of cases.[15] Cardiac computed tomography (CT) and MRI are the best imaging modalities for detecting an increase in pericardial thickness (>3 mm).[16] However, in as many as 20% of patients with surgically confirmed constrictive pericarditis, CT and MRI will demonstrate a pericardium of normal thickness.[17]

When faced with the diagnostic conundrum of constrictive pericarditis versus restrictive cardiomyopathy, strong clinical suspicion, thorough echocardiography, careful hemodynamic assessment with right and left heart catheterization,[14,18] pericardial imaging, and sometimes endomyocardial biopsy to exclude restrictive cardiomyopathy are often needed before proceeding to pericardiectomy, which carries a significant surgical risk but can also be curative.

This case highlights many of the features of constrictive pericarditis, the challenges and delay in its diagnosis, and its occasional misdiagnosis as a chronic liver disease. Clinicians may recognize the typical combination of cirrhosis (or suspected cirrhosis), high SAAG ascites, and edema as characteristic of advanced intrinsic liver disease. However, they must not be seduced into immediate pattern recognition when contrary evidence—such as elevated neck veins, elevated ascitic total protein, or relatively preserved hepatic synthetic function—accompanies that picture. Under such circumstances, they must remember to think outside the box, or hypothetico-deductively, and bear in mind that the heart may be trapped inside a "box."

Key Points

1. Constrictive pericarditis is often unrecognized initially, resulting in delayed diagnosis. Patients typically present with nonspecific signs and symptoms of low cardiac output and progressive right-sided heart failure. Clinical suspicion is key to prompt diagnosis and pericardiectomy, which may be curative.
2. Distinguishing features in the presentation of cardiac or pericardial etiologies of ascites and cirrhosis include elevated neck veins, elevated ascitic protein content, relatively preserved hepatic synthetic function, and absence of the stigmata of end-stage liver disease.
3. Constrictive pericarditis and restrictive cardiomyopathy can present with a similar clinical picture and hemodynamics showing impaired ventricular filling. Right and left heart catheterization, pericardial imaging, and endomyocardial biopsy may differentiate the two conditions. For constrictive pericarditis, surgical and pathological confirmation is the gold standard for diagnosis and the only definitive treatment.

REFERENCES

1. Ling LH, Oh JK, Schaff HV, et al. Constrictive pericarditis in the modern era: evolving clinical spectrum and impact on outcome after pericardiectomy. *Circulation*. 1999;100:1380–1386.
2. Bertog SC, Thambidorai SK, Parakh K, et al. Constrictive pericarditis: Etiology and cause-specific survival after pericardiectomy. *J Am Coll Cardiol*. 2004;43:1445–1452.
3. Wood P. Chronic constrictive pericarditis. *Am J Cardiol*. 1961;7:48–61.
4. American Gastroenterological Association. AGA technical review on the evaluation of liver chemistry tests. *Gastroenterology*. 2002;123:1367–1384.
5. Murray KF, Carithers RI. AASLD practice guidelines: Evaluation of the patient for liver transplantation. *Hepatology*. 2005;41:1–26.
6. Feldman M, Friedman LS, Brandt LJ, eds. *Sleisenger and Fordtran's Gastrointestinal and Liver Disease: Pathophysiology, Diagnosis, Management*. Philadelphia: Saunders Elsevier; 2006.
7. Summerskill WH, Davidson CS, Dible JH, et al. Cirrhosis of the liver: A study of alcoholic and nonalcoholic patients in Boston and London. *N Engl J Med*. 1960;261:1–9.
8. Charlton MR, Kondo M, Roberts SK, et al. Liver transplantation for cryptogenic cirrhosis. *Liver Transpl Surg*. 1997;3:359–364.
9. Nashchitz JE, Slobodin G, Lewis RJ, et al. Heart diseases affecting the liver and liver disease affecting the heart. *Am Heart J*. 2000;140:111–120.
10. Giallourakis CC, Rosenberg PM, Friedman LS. The liver in heart failure. *Clin Liver Dis*. 2002;6:947–967.
11. Laleman W, Van Landeghem L, Wilmer A, et al. Portal hypertension: From pathophysiology to clinical practice. *Liver Int*. 2005;25:1079–1090.
12. Garcia-Tsao G. Portal hypertension. *Curr Opin Gastroenterol*. 2006;22:254–262.
13. Guazzi M, Polese A, Magrini F, et al. Negative influences of ascites on the cardiac function of cirrhotic patients. *Am J Med*. 1975;59:165–170.
14. Nishimura RA. Constrictive pericarditis in the modern era: A diagnostic dilemma. *Heart*. 2001;86:619–623.
15. Ling LH, Oh JK, Tei C, et al. Calcific constrictive pericarditis: Is it still with us? *Ann Intern Med*. 2000;132:444–450.
16. Wang ZF, Reddy GP, Gotway MB, Yeh BM, Hetts SW, Higgins CB. CT and MR imaging of pericardial disease. *RadioGraphics*. 2003;23:S167–S180.
17. Talreja DR, Edwards WD, Danielson GK, et al. Constrictive pericarditis in 26 patients with histologically normal pericardial thickness. *Circulation*. 2003;108:1852–1857.
18. Hurrell DG, Nishimura RA, Higano ST, et al. Value of dynamic respiratory changes in left and right ventricular pressures for the diagnosis of constrictive pericarditis. *Circulation*. 1996;93:2007–2013.

CHAPTER 12

ARE WE THERE YET?

LISA H. WILLIAMS and GREGORY J. RAUGI
Primary and Specialty Medicine Service, Veterans Affairs Puget Sound Health Care System, Department of Medicine, The University of Washington School of Medicine, Seattle, Washington

GURPREET DHALIWAL
Department of Medicine, University of California, San Francisco, California; Medical Service, San Francisco VA Medical Center, San Francisco, California

SANJAY SAINT
Department of Internal Medicine, University of Michigan, Ann Arbor, Michigan; Ann Arbor VA Health Services Research and Development Field Program, Ann Arbor, Michigan; Patient Safety Enhancement Program, University of Michigan Health System, Ann Arbor, Michigan; Tuscan-American Safety Collaborative, Florence, Italy

BENJAMIN A. LIPSKY
Primary and Specialty Medicine Service, Veterans Affairs Puget Sound Health Care System, Department of Medicine, The University of Washington School of Medicine, Seattle, Washington

A 62-year-old man with psoriasis for more than 30 years presented to the emergency department with a scaly, pruritic rash involving his face, trunk, and extremities that he had had for the past 10 days. The rash was spreading and not responding to application of clobetasol ointment, which had helped his psoriasis in the past. He also reported mild pharyngitis, headache, and myalgias.

A patient with a chronic skin condition presenting with a new rash means the clinician must consider whether it is an alternative manifestation of the chronic disorder or a new illness. Psoriasis takes many forms including guttate psoriasis, which presents with small, droplike plaques and frequently follows respiratory infections (particularly those caused by *Streptococcus*). Well-controlled psoriasis rarely transforms after three decades, so I would consider other conditions. The tempo of illness makes certain life-threatening syndromes, including Stevens–Johnson syndrome, toxic shock syndrome, and purpura fulminans, unlikely. An allergic reaction, atopic dermatitis, or medication reaction is possible. Infections, either systemic (e.g., syphilis) or dermatologic (e.g., scabies), should be considered. Photosensitivity could involve the sun-exposed areas, such as the extremities and face. Seborrheic dermatitis can cause scaling lesions of the face and trunk but not the extremities. Vasculitis merits consideration, but dependent regions are typically affected more than the head. Mycosis fungoides or a paraneoplastic phenomenon could cause a diffuse rash in this age group.

Clinical Care Conundrums: Challenging Diagnoses in Hospital Medicine, First Edition.
Edited by James C. Pile, Thomas E. Baudendistel, and Brian J. Harte.

The patient had diabetes mellitus, hypertension, diverticulosis, and depression. Three months before, he had undergone surgical drainage of a perirectal abscess. His usual medications were lovastatin, paroxetine, insulin, hydrochlorothiazide, and lisinopril. Three weeks previously, he had completed a 10-day course of trimethoprim/sulfamethoxazole for an upper respiratory infection. Otherwise, he was taking no new medications. He was allergic to penicillin. He denied substance abuse, recent travel, or risk factors for human immunodeficiency virus (HIV) infection. He worked as an automobile painter, lived with his wife, and had a pet dog.

Physical examination revealed a well-appearing man with normal vital signs. His skin had well-defined circumscribed pink plaques, mostly 1–2 cm in size, with thick, silvery scales in the ears and on the dorsal and ventral arms and legs, chest, back, face, and scalp. There were no pustules or other signs of infection (Figs. 12.1 and 12.2). The nails exhibited distal onycholysis, oil spots, and rare pits. His posterior pharynx was mildly erythematous. The results of cardiovascular, pulmonary, and abdominal examinations were normal.

Although other scaling skin conditions such as eczema, irritant dermatitis, or malignancy remain possible, his rash is most consistent with widespread psoriasis. I would consider immunological changes that may have caused a remarkably altered and more severe expression of his chronic disease, for example, recent steroid therapy or HIV

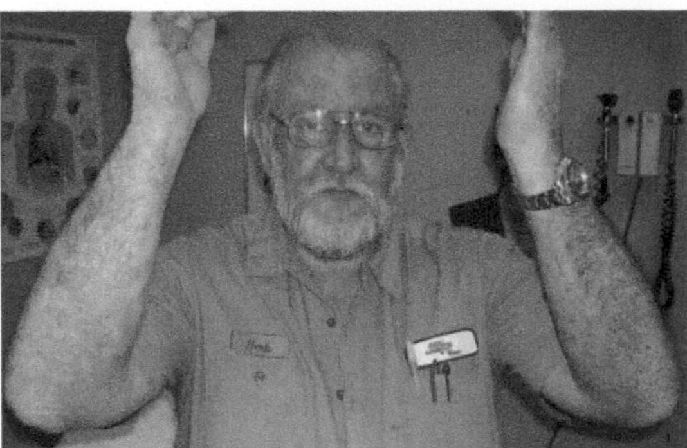

FIGURE 12.1 Circumscribed pink plaques with thick silvery scale on the extensor surfaces of arms and face.

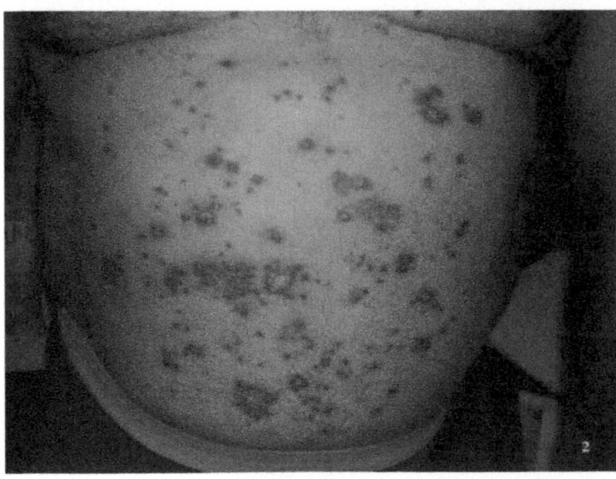

FIGURE 12.2 Similar plaques on abdomen, many with a guttate (droplike) pattern.

infection. The company a rash keeps helps frame the differential diagnosis. Based on the patient's well appearance, the time course, his minimal systemic symptoms, and the appearance of the rash, my leading considerations are psoriasis or an allergic dermatitis. Cutaneous T-cell malignancy, with its indolent and sometimes protean manifestations, remains possible in a patient of his age. I would now consult a dermatologist for three reasons: this patient has a chronic disease that I do not manage beyond basic treatments (eg, topical steroids), he has an undiagnosed illness with substantial dermatologic manifestations, and he may need a skin biopsy for definitive diagnosis.

The dermatology team diagnosed a guttate psoriasis flare, possibly associated with streptococcal pharyngitis. The differential diagnosis included secondary syphilis, although the team believed this was less likely. The dermatology team recommended obtaining a throat culture, streptozyme assay, and rapid plasma reagin and prescribed oral erythromycin and topical steroid ointment under a sauna suit.

I would follow his response to the prescribed steroid treatments. If the patient's course deviates from the dermatologists' expectations, I would request a skin biopsy and undertake further evaluations in search of an underlying systemic disease.

The patient followed up in the dermatology clinic 3 weeks later. His rash had worsened, and he had developed patchy alopecia and progressive edema of the face, ears, and eyes. He denied mouth or tongue swelling, difficulty breathing, or hives. The streptozyme assay was positive, but the other laboratory test results were negative.

The dermatology team diagnosed a severely inflammatory psoriasis flare and prescribed an oral retinoid, acitretin, and referred him for ultraviolet light therapy. He was unable to travel for phototherapy, and acitretin was discontinued after 1 week because of elevated serum transaminase levels. The dermatologists then prescribed oral cyclosporine.

The progression of disease despite standard treatment suggests a nonpsoriatic condition. Although medications could cause the abnormal liver tests, so could another underlying illness that involves the liver. An infiltrative disorder of the skin with hair follicle destruction and local lymphedema could explain both alopecia and facial edema.

I am unable account for his clinical features with a single disease, so the differential remains broad, including severe psoriasis, an infiltrating cutaneous malignancy, or a toxic exposure. Arsenic poisoning causes hyperkeratotic skin lesions, although he lacks the associated gastrointestinal and neurological symptoms. I would not have added the potentially toxic cyclosporine.

When he returned to dermatology clinic 1 week later, his rash and facial swelling had worsened. He also reported muscle and joint aches, fatigue, lightheadedness, anorexia, nausea, abdominal pain, diarrhea, and dyspnea on exertion. He denied fever, chills, and night sweats.

He appeared ill and used a cane to arise and walk. His vital signs and oxygen saturation were normal. He had marked swelling of his face, diffuse erythema and swelling on the chest, and widespread scaly, erythematous plaques (Fig. 12.3). The proximal nail folds of his fingers were erythematous, with ragged cuticles. His abdomen was mildly distended, but the rest of the physical examination was normal.

He has become too systemically ill to attribute his condition to psoriasis. The nail findings suggest dermatomyositis, which could explain many of his findings. The diffuse erythema and his difficulty walking are consistent with his skin and muscle involvement. Dyspnea could be explained by dermatomyositis-associated interstitial lung

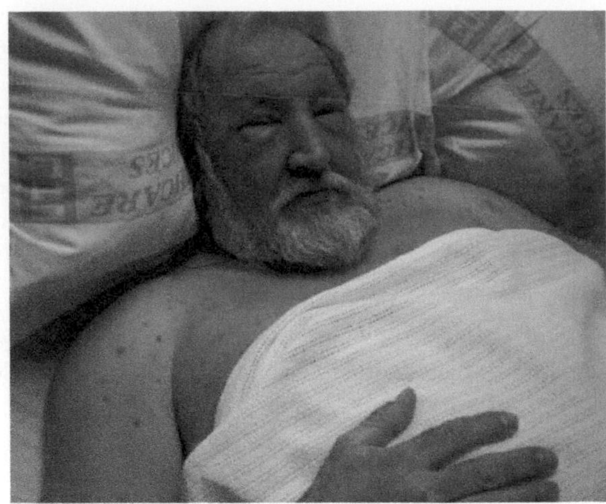

FIGURE 12.3 About 4 weeks later, there are erythematous plaques and marked swelling of the face, diffuse erythema and swelling of the chest, and persistent plaques on the arms and dorsal hands.

disease. A dermatomyositis-associated hematological or solid malignancy could account for his multisystem ailments and functional decline. A point against dermatomyositis is the relatively explosive onset of his disease. He should be carefully examined for any motor weakness. With his progressive erythroderma, I am also concerned about an advancing cutaneous T-cell lymphoma (with leukemic transformation).

Blood tests revealed the following values: white blood cell count, 8700/L; hematocrit, 46%; platelet count, 172,000/L; blood urea nitrogen, 26 mg/dL; creatinine, 1.0 mg/dL; glucose, 199 mg/dL; albumin, 3.1 g/dL; alkaline phosphatase, 172 U/L (normal range, 45–129); alanine aminotransferase, 75 U/L (normal range, 0–39 U/L); aspartate aminotransferase, 263 U/L (normal range, 0–37 U/L); total bilirubin, 1.1 mg/dL; prothrombin time, 16 seconds (normal range, 11.7–14.3 seconds); and serum creatinine kinase, 4253 U/L (normal range, 0–194 U/L). HIV serology was negative. Urinalysis revealed trace protein. The results of chest radiographs and an electrocardiogram were normal.

The liver function test results are consistent with medication effects or liver involvement in a systemic disease. The creatinine kinase elevation is consistent with a myopathy such as dermatomyositis. A skin biopsy would still be useful. Depending on those results, he may need a muscle biopsy, urine heavy metal testing, and computed tomography body imaging. Considering his transaminase and creatinine kinase elevations, I would discontinue lovastatin.

The patient was hospitalized. Further questioning revealed that he had typical Raynaud's phenomenon and odynophagia. A detailed neurological examination showed weakness (3/5) of the triceps and iliopsoas muscles and difficulty rising from a chair without using his arms. Dermatoscopic examination of the proximal nail folds showed dilated capillary loops and foci of hemorrhage.

Blood tests showed a lactate dehydrogenase level of 456 U/L (normal range, 0–249 U/L) and an aldolase of 38 U/L (normal range, 1.2–7.6 U/L). Tests for antinuclear antibodies, anti-Jo antibody, and antimyeloperoxidase antibodies were negative. Two skin biopsies were interpreted by general pathology as consistent with partially treated psoriasis, whereas another showed nonspecific changes with

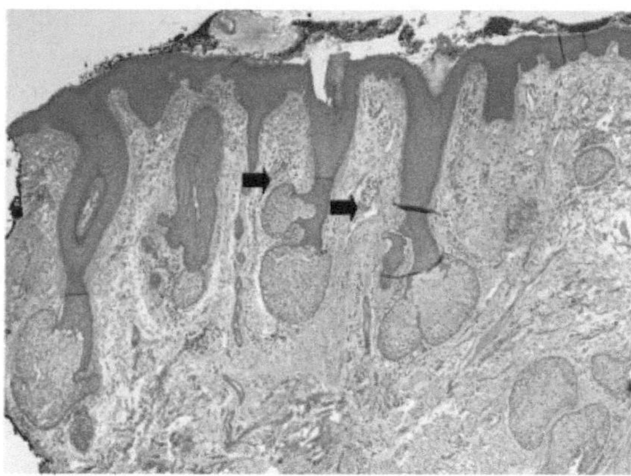

FIGURE 12.4 Photomicrograph of biopsy specimen of forehead skin showing superficial perivascular lymphohistiocytic inflammation (arrows).

minimal superficial perivascular lymphohistiocytic inflammation (Fig. 12.4). Lisinopril was discontinued because of its possible contribution to the facial edema.

Dermatomyositis is now the leading diagnosis. Characteristic features include his proximal muscle weakness, Raynaud's phenomenon, and dilated nail fold capillary loops. I am not overly dissuaded by the negative antinuclear antibodies, but because of additional atypical features (ie, extensive cutaneous edema, rapid onset, illness severity, prominent gastrointestinal symptoms), a confirmatory muscle biopsy is needed. Endoscopy of the proximal aerodigestive tract would help evaluate the odynophagia. There is little to suggest infection, malignancy, or metabolic derangement.

The inpatient medical team considered myositis related to retinoid or cyclosporine therapy. They discontinued cyclosporine and began systemic corticosteroid therapy. Within a few days, the patient's rash, muscle pain, and weakness improved, and the elevated transaminase and creatinine kinase levels decreased.

Dermatology recommended an evaluation for dermatomyositis-associated malignancy, but the medicine team and rheumatology consultants, noting the lack of classic skin findings (heliotrope rash and Gottron's papules) and the uncharacteristically rapid onset and improvement of myositis, suggested delaying the evaluation until dermatomyositis was proven.

An immediate improvement in symptoms with steroids is nonspecific, often occurring in autoimmune, infectious, and neoplastic diseases. This juncture in the case is common in complex multisystem illnesses, where various consultants may arrive at differing conclusions. With both typical and atypical features of dermatomyositis, where should one set the therapeutic threshold, that is, the point where one ends testing, accepts a diagnosis, and initiates treatment? Several factors raise the level of certainty I would require. First, dermatomyositis is quite rare. Adding atypical features further increases the burden of proof for that illness. Second, the existence of alternative possibilities (admittedly of equal uncertainty) gives me some pause. Finally, the toxicity of the proposed treatments raises the therapeutic threshold. Acknowledging that empiric treatment may be indicated for a severely ill patient at a lower level of certainty, I would hesitate to commit a patient to long-term steroids without being confident of the diagnosis. I would therefore require a muscle biopsy, or at least electromyography, to support or exclude dermatomyositis.

The patient was discharged from the hospital on high-dose prednisone. He underwent electromyography, which revealed inflammatory myopathic changes more apparent in the proximal than distal muscles. These findings were thought to be compatible with dermatomyositis, although the fibrillations and positive sharp waves characteristic of acute inflammation were absent, perhaps because of corticosteroid therapy.

The patient mistakenly stopped taking his prednisone. Within days, his weakness and skin rash worsened, and he developed nausea with vomiting. He returned to clinic, where his creatinine kinase level was again found to be elevated, and he was rehospitalized. Oral corticosteroid therapy was restarted with prompt improvement. On review of the original skin biopsies, a dermatopathologist observed areas of thickened dermal collagen and a superficial and deep perivascular lymphocytic infiltrate, both consistent with connective tissue disease.

These three additional findings (i.e., electromyography results, temporally established steroid responsiveness, and the new skin biopsy interpretation) in aggregate support the diagnosis of dermatomyositis, but the nausea and vomiting are unusual. I would discuss these results with a rheumatologist and still request a confirmatory muscle biopsy. Because diagnosing dermatomyositis should prompt consideration of seeking an underlying malignancy in a patient of this age group, I would repeat a targeted history and physical examination along with age- and risk-factor-appropriate screening. If muscle biopsy results are not definitive, finding an underlying malignancy would lend support to dermatomyositis.

While hospitalized, the patient complained of continued odynophagia and was noted to have oral candidiasis. Upper endoscopy, undertaken to evaluate for esophageal candidiasis, revealed a mass at the gastroesophageal junction. Biopsy revealed gastric-type adenocarcinoma. An abdominal computed tomography scan demonstrated three hypodense hepatic lesions, evidence of cirrhosis, and ascites. Cytology of paracentesis fluid revealed cells compatible with adenocarcinoma. The patient died in hospice care 2 weeks later.

At autopsy, he had metastatic gastric-type adenocarcinoma. A muscle biopsy (Fig. 12.5) revealed muscle atrophy with small foci of lymphocytic infiltrates, most compatible with dermatomyositis. Another dermatopathologist reviewed the skin

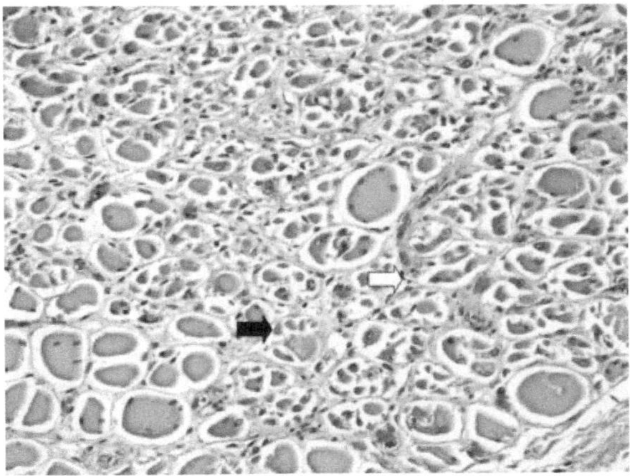

FIGURE 12.5 Biopsy specimen of the pectoralis major muscle showing extensive atrophy of muscle fibers (black arrow) with small foci of lymphocytic infiltrates (white arrow).

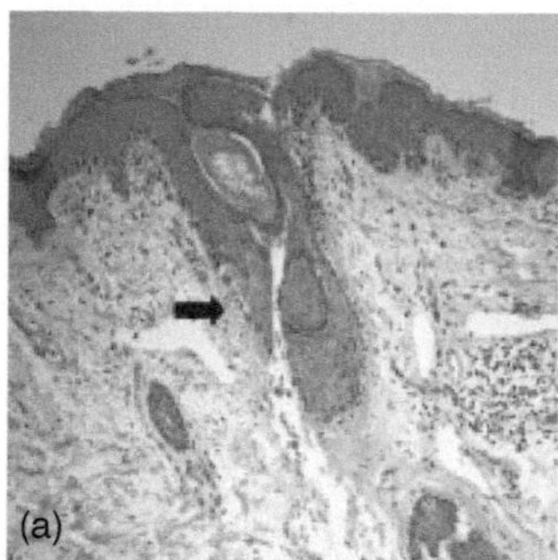

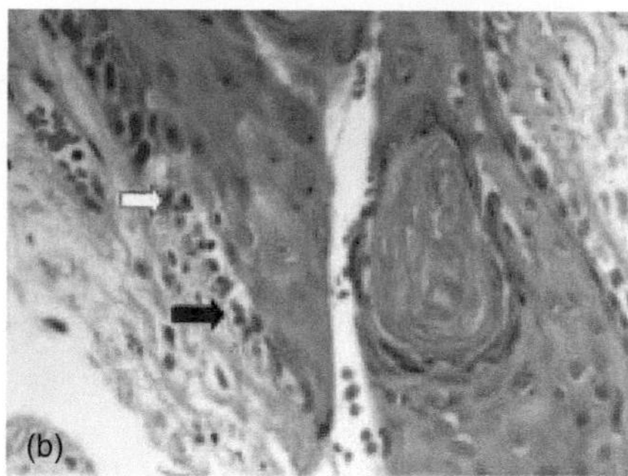

FIGURE 12.6 Biopsy specimen of (a) forehead skin showing characteristic interface dermatitis of a connective tissue disorder in a hair follicle. Mild lymphocytic inflammation and vacuolar changes at the dermoepidermal junction (black arrows), with (b) enlarged image showing dyskeratotic or degenerating keratinocytes (white arrow).

biopsies and noted interface dermatitis, which is typical of connective tissue diseases such as dermatomyositis (Fig. 12.6a,b).

COMMENTARY

Dermatomyositis is an idiopathic inflammatory myopathy characterized by endomysial inflammation and muscle weakness and differentiated from other myopathies by the presence of a rash.[1] Muscle disease may manifest with or precede the rash, but up to 40% of patients present with skin manifestations alone, an entity called *amyopathic dermatomyositis*.[2] When present, the myositis generally develops over months, but the onset can be acute.[1] The weakness is typically symmetrical and proximal,[1] and many patients have oropharyngeal dysphagia.[3]

The characteristic rash is erythematous, symmetrical, and photodistributed.[4] Classic cutaneous findings are the heliotrope rash (violaceous eyelid erythema), which is pathognomonic but uncommon, and the more common Gottron's papules (violaceous, slightly elevated papules and plaques on bony prominences and extensor surfaces, especially the knuckles).[4] Other findings include periorbital edema, scalp dermatitis, poikiloderma (ie, hyperpigmentation, hypopigmentation, atrophy, and telangiectasia), periungual erythema, and dystrophic cuticles.[2] The cutaneous manifestations of dermatomyositis may be similar to those of psoriasis, systemic lupus erythematosus, lichen planus, rosacea, polymorphous light eruption, drug eruption, atopic dermatitis, seborrheic dermatitis, or allergic contact dermatitis.[4]

Diagnosing dermatomyositis requires considering clinical, laboratory, electromyographical, and histological evidence, as there are no widely accepted, validated diagnostic criteria.[1,5] The diagnosis is usually suspected if there is a characteristic rash and symptoms of myositis (eg, proximal muscle weakness, myalgias, fatigue, or an inability to swallow). When the patient has an atypical rash, skin biopsy can differentiate dermatomyositis from other conditions, except lupus, which shares the key finding of interface dermatitis.[2] The histological findings can be variable and subtle,[6] so consultation with a dermatopathologist may be helpful.

Myositis may be confirmed by various studies. Most patients have elevated muscle enzymes (ie, creatinine kinase, aldolase, lactate dehydrogenase, or transaminases)[1]; for those who do not, magnetic resonance imaging can be helpful in detecting muscle involvement and locating the best site for muscle biopsy.[7] Electromyography reveals nonspecific muscle membrane instability.[8] Muscle biopsy shows muscle fiber necrosis, perifascicular atrophy, and perivascular and perifascicular lymphocytic infiltrates. These can be patchy, diminished by steroid use, and occasionally seen in noninflammatory muscular dystrophies.[8] For a patient with typical myositis and a characteristic rash, muscle biopsy may be unnecessary.[1]

The clinical utility of serologic testing for diagnosing dermatomyositis is controversial.[2] Myositis-specific antibody testing is insensitive but specific; these antibodies include Jo-1, an antisynthetase antibody that predicts incomplete response to therapy and lung involvement, and Mi-2, which is associated with better response to therapy.[2,9,10] The sensitivity and specificity of antinuclear antibodies are both approximately 60%.[10]

Patients with dermatomyositis have higher rates of cancers than age-matched controls, and nearly 25% of patients are diagnosed with a malignancy at some point during the course of the disease.[11] Malignancies are typically solid tumors that manifest within 3 years of the diagnosis,[12–14] although the increased risk may exist for at least 5 years.[14] There is a 10-fold higher risk of ovarian cancer in women with dermatomyositis.[12,15] Other associated malignancies include lung, gastric, colorectal, pancreatic, and breast carcinomas and non-Hodgkin's lymphoma.[14]

Recommendations for screening affected patients for cancer have changed over the years, with increasing evidence of an association between dermatomyositis and malignancy and evolving improvements in diagnostic techniques.[16] Many authorities recommend that all adult patients with dermatomyositis be evaluated for cancer, including a complete physical examination, basic hematological tests, age- and sex-appropriate screening (e.g., mammography, pap smear, and colonoscopy), and chest X-ray.[16] Some would add upper endoscopy; imaging of the chest, abdomen, and pelvis; gynecological examination; and serum CA-125 level to better evaluate for the most common malignancies (i.e., ovarian, gastric, lung, and pancreatic carcinomas and non-Hodgkin's lymphoma).[12,17–20]

In 19% of adults, dermatomyositis overlaps with other autoimmune disorders, usually systemic lupus erythematosus and systemic sclerosis.[21] These manifest as Raynaud's phenomenon, arthritis, esophageal dysmotility, renal disease, or neuropathy.[21] Other potentially serious systemic manifestations of dermatomyositis include proximal dysphagia from pharyngeal myopathy; distal dysphagia from esophageal dysmotility in systemic sclerosis overlap; pulmonary disease from autoimmune interstitial lung disease or aspiration; cardiac disease from conduction abnormalities, myocarditis, pericarditis, and valvular disease; and rhabdomyolysis.[2]

Treatment of dermatomyositis requires systemic immunosuppression with one or more agents. The prognosis of dermatomyositis is variable. Mortality at 5 years ranges from 23% to 73%. At least one-third of patients are left with mild to severe disability.[1] In addition to older age, predictors of poor outcome include male sex, dysphagia, longstanding symptoms before treatment, pulmonary or cardiac involvement, and presence of antisynthetase antibodies.[22]

Dermatomyositis is often treated in the outpatient setting, but there are many reasons for hospitalization. Complications of treatment, such as infection or adverse effects of medications, could result in hospitalization. Treatment with intravenous pulse corticosteroids or IVIG may require inpatient administration if no infusion center is available. Other indications for inpatient evaluation include the consequences of various malignancies and the more severe expression of systemic complications of dermatomyositis (e.g., dysphagia and pulmonary, cardiac, or renal disease).

Every parent knows the plaintive backseat whine, "Are we *there*, yet?" Clinicians may also experience this feeling when attempting to diagnose a perplexing illness, especially one that lacks a definitive diagnostic test. It was easy for this patient's doctors to assume initially that his new rash was a manifestation of his long-standing psoriasis. Having done so, they could understandably attribute the subsequent findings to either evolution of this disease or to consequences of the prescribed treatments, rather than considering a novel diagnosis. Only when faced with new (or newly appreciated) findings suggesting myopathy, the clinicians (and our discussant) considered the diagnosis of dermatomyositis. Even then, the primary inpatient medical team and their consultants were unsure when they had sufficient evidence to be certain.

Several factors compounded the difficulty of making a diagnosis in this case: the clinicians were dealing with a rare disease, they were considering alternative diagnoses (ie, psoriasis or a toxic effect of medication), and the disease presented somewhat atypically. The clinicians initially failed to consider and then accept the correct diagnosis because the patient's rash was not classic, his biopsy was interpreted as nonspecific, and he lacked myositis at presentation. Furthermore, when the generalists sought expert assistance, they encountered a difference of opinion among the consultants. These complex situations should goad the clinician into carefully considering the therapeutic threshold, that is, the transition point from diagnostic testing to therapeutic intervention.[23] With complex cases like this, it may be difficult to know when one has reached an adequately supported diagnosis, and frequently asking whether we are "there" yet may be appropriate.

Key Points

1. The diagnosis of dermatomyositis may be challenging, given the absence of a "gold standard" test. A combination of clinical, laboratory, biopsy, and electromyographic data may need to be considered to arrive at the diagnosis.
2. Ovarian, lung, gastric, colorectal, pancreatic, and breast carcinomas, as well as non-Hodgkin's lymphoma, are the most common cancers associated with dermatomyositis. In addition to age-appropriate cancer screening, one should consider obtaining upper endoscopy, imaging chest/abdomen/pelvis, and a serum CA-125 test in these patients.
3. Patients with dermatomyositis and no obvious concurrent malignancy need long-term outpatient follow-up for repeated malignancy screening.

REFERENCES

1. Dalakas MC, Hohlfeld R. Polymyositis and dermatomyositis. *Lancet*. 2003;362:971–982.
2. Callen JP. Dermatomyositis. *Lancet*. 2000;355:53–47.
3. Ertekin C, Secil Y, Yuceyar N, Aydogdu I. Oropharyngeal dysphagia in polymyositis/dermatomyositis. *Clin Neurol Neurosurg*. 2004;107(1):32–37.
4. Santmyire-Rosenberger B, Dugan EM. Skin involvement in dermatomyositis. *Curr Opin Rheumatol*. 2003;15:714–22.
5. Troyanov Y, Targoff IN, Tremblay JL, Goulet JR, Raymond Y, Senecal JL. Novel classification of idiopathic inflammatory myopathies based on overlap syndrome features and auto-antibodies: Analysis of 100 French Canadian patients. *Medicine (Baltimore)*. 2005;84:231–249.
6. Weedon D. *Skin pathology*. 2nd ed. New York: Churchill Livingstone; 2002.
7. Park JH, Olsen NJ. Utility of magnetic resonance imaging in the evaluation of patients with inflammatory myopathies. *Curr Rheumatol Rep*. 2001;3:334–245.
8. Nirmalananthan N, Holton JL, Hanna MG. Is it really myositis? A consideration of the differential diagnosis. *Curr Opin Rheumatol*. 2004;16:684–691.

9. Targoff IN. Idiopathic inflammatory myopathy: Autoantibody update. *Curr Rheumatol Rep*. 2002;4: 434–441.
10. van Paassen P, Damoiseaux J, Tervaert JW. Laboratory assessment in musculoskeletal disorders. *Best Pract Res Clin Rheumatol*. 2003;17:475–494.
11. Callen JP, Wortmann RL. Dermatomyositis. *Clin Dermatol*. 2006;24:363–373.
12. Hill CL, Zhang Y, Sigurgeirsson B, et al. Frequency of specific cancer types in dermatomyositis and polymyositis: A population-based study. *Lancet*. 2001;357:96–100.
13. Ponyi A, Constantin T, Garami M, et al. Cancer-associated myositis: Clinical features and prognostic signs. *Ann NY Acad Sci*. 2005;1051:64–71.
14. Buchbinder R, Forbes A, Hall S, Dennett X, Giles G. Incidence of malignant disease in biopsy-proven inflammatory myopathy. A population-based cohort study. *Ann Intern Med*. 2001;134:1087–1095.
15. Stockton D, Doherty VR, Brewster DH. Risk of cancer in patients with dermatomyositis or polymyositis, and follow-up implications: A Scottish population-based cohort study. *Br J Cancer*. 2001;85(1):41–45.
16. Callen JP. When and how should the patient with dermatomyositis or amyopathic dermatomyositis be assessed for possible cancer? *Arch Dermatol*. 2002;138:969–971.
17. Whitmore SE, Rosenshein NB, Provost TT. Ovarian cancer in patients with dermatomyositis. *Medicine (Baltimore)*. 1994;73(3):153–160.
18. Whitmore SE, Watson R, Rosenshein NB, Provost TT. Dermatomyositis sine myositis: Association with malignancy. *J Rheumatol*. 1996;23(1):101–105.
19. Amoura Z, Duhaut P, Huong DL, et al. Tumor antigen markers for the detection of solid cancers in inflammatory myopathies. *Cancer Epidemiol Biomarkers Prev*. 2005;14:1279–1282.
20. Sparsa A, Liozon E, Herrmann F, et al. Routine vs extensive malignancy search for adult dermatomyositis and polymyositis: A study of 40 patients. *Arch Dermatol*. 2002;138:885–890.
21. Dawkins MA, Jorizzo JL, Walker FO, Albertson D, Sinal SH, Hinds A. Dermatomyositis: A dermatology-based case series. *J Am Acad Dermatol*. 1998;38:397–404.
22. Bronner IM, van der Meulen MF, de Visser M, et al. Long-term outcome in polymyositis and dermatomyositis. *Ann Rheum Dis*. 2006;65:1456–1461.
23. Kassirer JP. Our stubborn quest for diagnostic certainty. A cause of excessive testing. *N Engl J Med*. 1989;320:1489–1491.

CHAPTER **13**

A DISTINGUISHING FEATURE

SANJIV J. SHAH
Department of Medicine, University of Chicago, Chicago, Illinois; Department of Medicine, University of California, San Francisco, California

AUBREY O. INGRAHAM
Department of Medicine, Kaiser Permanente Medical Center, Oakland, California

SANDRA Y. CHUNG
Department of Medicine, University of California, San Francisco, California

RICHARD J. HABER
Department of Medicine, University of California, San Francisco, California; Department of Medicine, San Francisco General Hospital, San Francisco, California

A 56-year-old man with a history of chronic liver disease of unknown etiology was referred to a tertiary care center for evaluation of intermittent low-grade fevers, constipation, and an unintentional weight loss of 20 kg during the previous 9 months. Three weeks prior to presentation, he was admitted to his local hospital for these symptoms and was treated empirically with cefotaxime for 6 days, but his symptoms persisted.

The patient's age and sex make him statistically at risk for vascular disease as well as malignancy. The history of chronic liver disease of unknown etiology is intriguing. In evaluating a patient with chronic liver disease, critical features of the history include alcohol consumption, intravenous drug use, family history, viral hepatitis serology, and any known antinuclear antibody testing. Chronic liver disease places this patient at increased risk for infection because portal hypertension causes blood to bypass a large part of the reticuloendothelial system (liver and spleen), therefore increasing the risk of sustained bacteremia.

Regarding his chronic low-grade fever, I would like to know about his country of origin, travel history, occupational history, risk factors for human immunodeficiency virus (HIV) and tuberculosis, and any symptoms or signs of rheumatologic disease. Constipation and weight loss can be a result of malignancy (e.g., hepatocellular carcinoma, colorectal cancer), vascular disease (e.g., mesenteric thrombosis), or metabolic derangement (e.g., hypercalcemia).

The patient had a history of recurrent episodes of ascites and low-grade fevers. He first developed ascites, abdominal pain, low-grade fevers, and pedal edema 20 years ago. These signs and symptoms resolved spontaneously, but similar episodes

Clinical Care Conundrums: Challenging Diagnoses in Hospital Medicine, First Edition.
Edited by James C. Pile, Thomas E. Baudendistel, and Brian J. Harte.

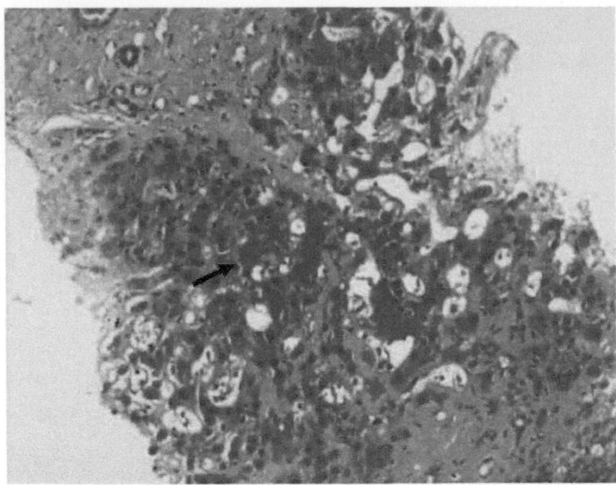

FIGURE 13.1 Liver biopsy specimen showing extensive scarring (arrow) interspersed with areas of completely normal liver parenchyma (hematoxylin and eosin, X400).

have recurred every 4–6 years since. Each time, diagnostic evaluation failed to reveal a specific etiology.

Twelve years prior to presentation, the patient was evaluated for chronic liver disease. Diagnostic tests at that time included viral hepatitis serology, ceruloplasmin, ferritin, alpha-1-antitrypsin, antimitochondrial antibody, and antinuclear antibody testing, all the results of which were within the normal range. The patient denied consumption of alcohol, medications, or toxic substances. Percutaneous liver biopsy demonstrated focal parenchymal scarring interspersed with areas of normal parenchyma, consistent with focal ischemic injury (Fig. 13.1).

The duration of the patient's symptoms is striking. A unifying diagnosis for this patient must explain his chronic liver disease, periodic fevers, ascites, and abdominal pain that started at a relatively young age. Conditions to consider include hepatitis B or C, hemochromatosis, Wilson's disease, primary biliary cirrhosis, primary sclerosing cholangitis, autoimmune hepatitis, alpha-1-antitrypsin deficiency, and drug or toxin exposure. Veno-occlusive disease of the liver and chronic congestive hepatopathy (from heart failure or constrictive pericarditis) are especially attractive possibilities, given the findings of focal ischemic injury on liver biopsy.

Recurrent fever and abdominal pain can occur because of familial Mediterranean fever, which results from a genetic abnormality and causes recurrent peritoneal inflammation associated with fever and ascites. Although unlikely in this case, familial Mediterranean fever can cause secondary amyloidosis with liver involvement.

The patient reported episodic vague abdominal pain, nausea, anorexia, night sweats, hair thinning, extreme fatigue, and lightheadedness. He had no known allergies, and his medications included propranolol, lactulose, docusate, and omeprazole. He was white, born in the United States, and a lawyer, but he had not worked during the previous 4 months. He was married and monogamous, and an HIV antibody test 4 months prior was negative. He had a remote history of tobacco and alcohol use between the 1960s and the 1980s. He denied intravenous drug use. His family history was only remarkable for a father with coronary artery disease.

With fever, the hypothalamic set point for temperature increases. Night sweats usually indicate an exaggeration of the normal diurnal drop in the hypothalamic set point for temperature, with dissipation of increased heat (caused by fever) through evaporation of perspiration. Unfortunately, night sweats are not specific to any particular cause of fever.

Fatigue is equally nonspecific but could result from anemia, hypothyroidism, or adrenal insufficiency or could be a side effect of the propranolol. The lack of a family history makes hereditary periodic fevers unlikely.

The patient appeared chronically ill. His temperature was 35.2°C; blood pressure, 71/53 mm Hg; heart rate, 84 beats per minute; respiratory rate, 14 breaths per minute; and oxygen saturation, 99% while breathing room air. His weight was 47 kg. Examination of the patient's head and neck revealed bitemporal wasting but no scleral icterus, and the oropharynx was clear. There was no thyromegaly or lymphadenopathy. Cardiopulmonary examination was normal. The abdomen was soft with mild diffuse tenderness. There was no organomegaly or obvious ascites. His extremities were warm and without edema or cyanosis. He was dark-skinned and had rare spider angiomas. His neurological examination was normal.

Sepsis, drug ingestion (particularly vasodilators), environmental exposure, and endocrine abnormalities such as adrenal insufficiency and hypothyroidism can all cause both hypothermia and hypotension. Adrenal insufficiency is especially intriguing because it is also associated with malaise, abdominal pain, and hyperpigmentation. Explaining both adrenal insufficiency and chronic liver disease is more difficult. Hemochromatosis can cause cirrhotic liver disease, adrenal and thyroid insufficiency, and dark skin, but the patient's normal ferritin and liver biopsy findings make this disease unlikely.

The results of the laboratory studies were white blood cell count, 4900/mm^3, with a normal differential count; hemoglobin, 11.0 g/dL; platelet count, 52,000/mm^3; mean corpuscular volume, 89 μm^3; sodium, 131 mmol/L; potassium, 5.0 mmol/L; chloride, 101 mmol/L; bicarbonate, 21 mmol/L; blood urea nitrogen, 31 mg/dL; creatinine, 1.8 mg/dL; aspartate aminotransferase, 45 U/L (normal range, 16–41 U/L); alanine aminotransferase, 30 U/L (normal range, 12–59 U/L); alkaline phosphatase, 587 U/L (normal range, 29–111 U/L); total bilirubin, 1.1 mg/dL (normal range, 0.3–1.3 mg/dL); gamma-glutamyl transferase, 169 U/L (normal range, 7–71 U/L); lactate dehydrogenase, 127 IU/L (normal range, 91–185 IU/L); and thyroid-stimulating hormone, 3.1 mIU/L (normal range, 0.5–4.7 mIU/L). Coagulation studies revealed a prothrombin time of 12 seconds [international normalized ratio (INR) 1.1] and an activated partial thromboplastin time (aPTT) of greater than 100 seconds. Urinalysis and chest radiography were unremarkable.

The low sodium, high potassium, and relatively low bicarbonate levels are all compatible with adrenal insufficiency. When present, the combination of hyponatremia (primarily from glucocorticoid deficiency) and hyperkalemia (from mineralocorticoid deficiency) suggests that the adrenal insufficiency is primary, rather than from the pituitary. The differential diagnosis of primary adrenal insufficiency includes autoimmune disease, granulomatous disease, and tumor.

Most interesting is the isolated prolongation of the aPTT, making adrenal hemorrhage another possibility as a cause of the adrenal insufficiency. Isolated elevation of the aPTT suggests deficiency or inhibition of the factors involved in the intrinsic pathway (factors VIII, IX, XI, and XII) or the presence of an antiphospholipid antibody, which would interfere with the test. Heparin administration (which may not be immediately obvious, as in the case of a heparin lock of an intravenous line) and von Willebrand disease (from loss of the normal von-Willebrand-factor-associated prevention of factor VIII proteolysis) can also cause isolated prolongation of the aPTT.

Tumor, perhaps hepatocellular cancer, remains a possible explanation for the elevated alkaline phosphatase, with possible adrenal involvement. Amyloidosis and diffuse granulomatous disease (either infectious or noninfectious, such as sarcoidosis) can cause elevation in alkaline phosphatase. At this time, I would rule out adrenal insufficiency, further evaluate the elevated aPTT, and image the liver and adrenal glands.

The patient was hospitalized and given intravenous fluids. His blood pressure increased to 90/54 mm Hg. Further testing revealed an alpha-fetoprotein of 1.5 μg/dL (normal range, <6.4 μg/dL), an erythrocyte sedimentation rate of greater than 100 mm/s, and normal results of an antinuclear antibody test. Serum cortisol, drawn at 6 am, was 3 ng/dL; 60 minutes after cosyntropin stimulation, serum cortisol was 1 ng/dL. An ultrasound of the liver revealed chronic hepatic vein thrombosis.

The low absolute values and the failure of serum cortisol to respond to cosyntropin confirm the diagnosis of adrenal glucocorticoid deficiency. Hepatic vein thrombosis (Budd–Chiari syndrome) is an unusual occurrence, often associated with a hypercoagulable state or tumor.

Primary antiphospholipid antibody syndrome is the most attractive unifying diagnosis because it appears to explain the most abnormalities with the fewest diagnoses. This syndrome includes arterial and venous thrombosis, thrombocytopenia, and isolated elevation of the aPTT and has been associated with hepatic vein thrombosis (acute and chronic) and adrenal insufficiency (from adrenal hemorrhage as a result of adrenal vein thrombosis). The histological findings of focal ischemic injury, seen on the patient's liver biopsy, are likely explained by hepatic veno-occlusive disease.

Magnetic resonance imaging (MRI) of the abdomen (Fig. 13.2) demonstrated adrenal hemorrhage in the right adrenal gland. The patient's aPTT remained elevated even after his serum was mixed with normal serum, and the results of the dilute Russell's viper venom time test also showed elevation. The addition of phospholipids to the patient's serum corrected the aPTT, and a screen for factor inhibitors was negative. An anticardiolipin antibody (IgG) test was positive at 59.0 U (normal, 0.4–2.3 U).

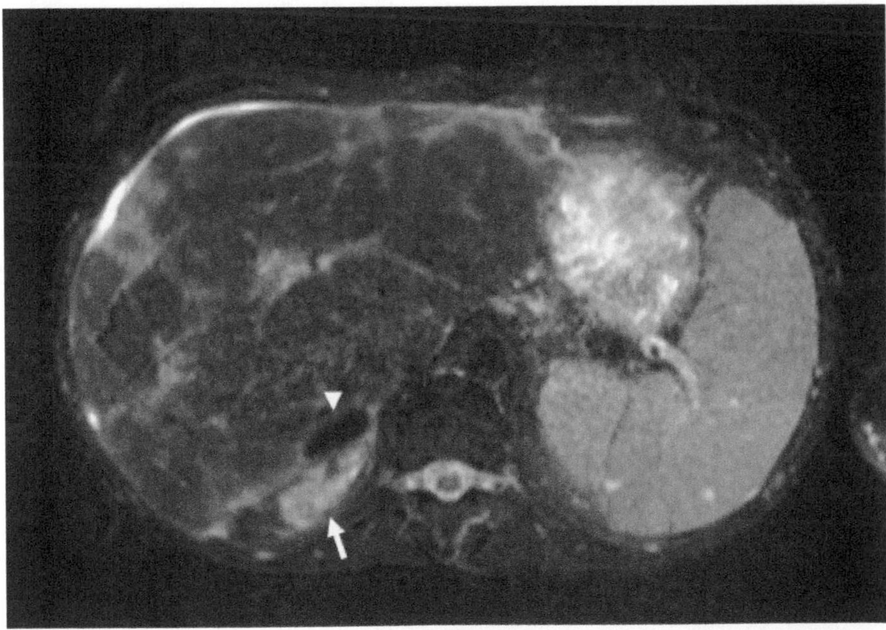

FIGURE 13.2 Magnetic resonance imaging of the abdomen showing right adrenal hemorrhage (arrow) adjacent to the inferior vena cava (arrowhead).

The findings of a bone marrow biopsy, performed to exclude infiltrative diseases, were normal. The patient was diagnosed with primary antiphospholipid syndrome. Hydrocortisone and fludrocortisone were initiated, with the intention to continue them indefinitely. The patient was also started on intravenous heparin, which continued until he achieved a goal INR of 2.0–3.0 on warfarin. The patient was counseled on the importance of lifelong warfarin therapy given his diagnosis of antiphospholipid syndrome with hepatic vein and adrenal vein thromboses. On follow-up 6 months after discharge, the patient's hypotension and fatigue had resolved, his alkaline phosphatase level had decreased substantially, and he had returned to work as a lawyer.

COMMENTARY

The diagnosis of a complex case with numerous clinical and laboratory abnormalities can be very difficult. The discussant successfully came to the correct diagnosis because he carefully evaluated each piece of evidence and did not fall prey to faulty "triggering," the generation of diagnostic hypotheses based on selected pieces of clinical data.[1] In the diagnostic process, physicians trigger new diagnostic possibilities and discard initial hypotheses as new findings emerge. Often, because of heuristic (analytic) biases, physicians fall victim to faulty triggering when evaluating patients.[2] When confronted with a "trigger feature" such as night sweats, many physicians increase their consideration of tuberculosis or lymphoma at the expense of more common diagnoses, even though, as the discussant pointed out, any patient with fever can have this symptom.[3] Whereas faulty use of trigger features may make physicians inappropriately consider uncommon diseases, a "distinguishing feature" limits the number of diagnostic possibilities and significantly changes—increases or decreases—the likelihood of there being a rare disease.[4] By correctly using the distinguishing feature of an elevated aPTT in the context of the patient's diverse clinical features, the discussant was able to arrive at a single unifying diagnosis of antiphospholipid syndrome.

Antiphospholipid syndrome is an arterial or a venous thrombosis associated with significantly elevated antiphospholipid antibodies. Isolated prolongation of the aPTT is often the first clue to the presence of antiphospholipid antibodies, which interfere with phospholipid-dependent coagulation assays.[5] Antiphospholipid syndrome is considered primary if it is not associated with a known underlying disease or medication. Antiphospholipid syndrome is secondary if it is associated with certain diseases such as systemic lupus erythematosus and malignancy or with an adverse effect of medication. Although the prevalence of antiphospholipid antibodies is 1%–5% in young, apparently healthy control subjects, it is higher in elderly patients with chronic diseases.[6] It remains unclear why only certain patients with antiphospholipid antibodies manifest the syndrome, although having vascular risk factors may increase the risk of developing thrombosis in the presence of antiphospholipid antibodies.[7]

Three types of antiphospholipid antibody tests are currently in clinical use: lupus anticoagulants (measured by prolonged clotting time in a phospholipid-dependent clotting test, such as the aPTT), anticardiolipin antibodies, and anti-β_2-glycoprotein I antibodies. All three tests are plagued by not being standardized between hospitals and laboratories and have limited sensitivity and specificity.[8,9] Lupus anticoagulants are most closely associated with thrombosis. Although a prolonged aPTT in the presence of thrombosis is often the first clue to the presence of lupus anticoagulants, only 30%–40% of patients with the syndrome have this laboratory abnormality.[10] Therefore, a normal aPTT result does not rule out the presence of antiphospholipid antibodies, and other tests of lupus anticoagulants, such as the dilute Russell viper venom time (which tests the phospholipid-dependent portion of the coagulation cascade), should be performed.[8,9] There are many types of anticardiolipin antibodies of varying immunoglobulin isotypes, which all share the ability to bind cardiolipin in vitro. The IgG isotypes (as in this patient) are thought to be most closely associated with thrombosis, and it is known that high titers of anti-cardiolipin antibodies have much better discriminatory value than low titers.[8–10] There is little data on the anti-β_2-glycoprotein I antibodies, but preliminary data suggest these antibodies may be more specific for the antiphospholipid syndrome.[11]

The antiphospholipid syndrome has classically been associated with lower-extremity deep venous thrombosis, recurrent fetal loss, thrombocytopenia, and livedo reticularis.[10] However, depending on the size and distribution of the vasculature involved and the extent and chronicity of involvement, the antiphospholipid syndrome can result in a wide range of manifestations. Acute presentations such as thrombotic disease of the gastrointestinal, cardiac, and central nervous systems can be rapid and catastrophic. A more chronic and indolent course can lead to progressive organ dysfunction, as in this patient, with chronic liver disease resulting from recurrent episodes of hepatic veno-occlusive disease and chronic hepatic vein thrombosis, a rare but well-described complication of antiphospholipid syndrome.[12,13] It is unclear why the course of this patient's hepatic vein thrombosis waxed and waned. One hypothesis is that he had episodes of microvascular hepatic venous thrombosis that led to transient hepatic dysfunction, with subsequent recovery upon spontaneous recanalization of hepatic veins or with healing and regeneration of liver tissue.

Treatment of antiphospholipid syndrome is controversial. Although prior reports suggested that patients with this syndrome were at higher risk for recurrent thrombosis when treated with the usual dose of warfarin (target INR, 2.0–3.0), two randomized trials showed there was no difference in the recurrence of thrombosis between moderate-intensity treatment with warfarin and high-intensity treatment with warfarin.[14,15] This patient was treated with warfarin to a moderate-intensity target INR of 2.0–3.0 because he had liver disease and adrenal hemorrhage.

Adrenal insufficiency is another rare complication of antiphospholipid syndrome. It was first described as such in 1980[16] and has been reported in both children and adults.[17–19] Abdominal pain and hypotension were the most common findings (55% and 54%, respectively) in one case series of 86 patients with adrenal insufficiency from antiphospholipid syndrome.[20] Fever, nausea, vomiting, weakness, fatigue, lethargy, and altered mental status were also variably present. Loss of adrenal function is most often a result of adrenal hemorrhage, which is best detected by MRI of the adrenal glands.[21]

The vascular anatomy of the adrenal gland is unusual. Multiple arteries supply the gland, but only one central vein provides drainage, making the gland relatively vulnerable to hemorrhagic infarction.[22] Most cases of adrenal insufficiency from antiphospholipid syndrome are thought to be a result of adrenal vein thrombosis. The MRI showed that only the right adrenal gland of this patient had evidence of hemorrhage. Because both adrenal glands must be damaged before adrenal insufficiency results, it is probable that the left adrenal gland was damaged because of prior episodes of infarction and/or hemorrhage, but remote damage could not be detected by MRI. Of note, antiphospholipid antibodies directed against cholesterol-rich proteins in the adrenal gland can also cause a locally active procoagulant state with microvascular venous thrombosis and subsequent postinfarction hemorrhage, which is another way in which the left adrenal gland could have been damaged without showing up radiographically.[23]

As for other types of adrenal insufficiency, the primary treatment for adrenal insufficiency from antiphospholipid syndrome is rapid corticosteroid replacement, with the addition of anticoagulants to treat the hypercoagulable state of the antiphospholipid syndrome. Adrenal insufficiency is temporary in some cases.[24] Mortality from adrenal insufficiency due to antiphospholipid syndrome may be higher than that from other forms of adrenal insufficiency.[22] Therefore, screening for adrenal insufficiency is critical for any patient with suspected or documented antiphospholipid syndrome who presents with abdominal pain, weakness, electrolyte abnormalities, or unexplained hypotension.

This case illustrates the importance, as the key to diagnosis, of determining a distinguishing feature such as a prolonged aPTT from among the multitude of abnormalities that could have led the diagnostic process astray. Occasionally, a single clinical or laboratory abnormality, such as the elevated aPTT in our patient, is so valuable in the assessment of a difficult case that it significantly increases the likelihood of an uncommon condition and leads to the correct final diagnosis, thereby becoming the pivotal "distinguishing feature."

Key Points

1. Hypercoagulability can lead to adrenal insufficiency by causing adrenal vein thrombosis and adrenal infarction. Therefore, hypercoagulable states, such as antiphospholipid syndrome, should be considered for patients who present with unexplained adrenal insufficiency.
2. Isolated elevation of aPTT suggests deficiency or inhibition of the factors involved in the intrinsic pathway (factors VIII, IX, XI, and XII) or the presence of an antiphospholipid antibody. Heparin administration and von Willebrand disease can also cause isolated prolongation of the aPTT.
3. Two recent trials suggest that patients with antiphospholipid syndrome who have had their first episode of thrombosis should be treated with warfarin, with a goal INR of 2.0–3.0.

REFERENCES

1. Kassirer JP. Diagnostic reasoning. *Ann Intern Med*. 1989;110:893–900.
2. Kassirer JP, Kopelman RI. Cognitive errors in diagnosis: Instantiation, classification, and consequences. *Am J Med*. 1989;86:433–441.
3. Viera AJ, Bond MM, Yates SW. Diagnosing night sweats. *Am Fam Physician*. 2003;67:1019–1024.
4. Smith CS, Paauw DS. When you hear hoof beats: Four principles for separating zebras from horses. *J Am Board Fam Pract*. 2000;13:424–429.
5. Levine JS, Branch DW, Rauch J. The antiphospholipid syndrome. *N Engl J Med*. 2002;346:752–763.
6. Petri M. Epidemiology of the antiphospholipid antibody syndrome. *J Autoimmun*. 2000;15:145–151.
7. Giron-Gonzalez JA, Garcia del Rio E, Rodriguez C, Rodriguez-Martorell J, Serrano A. Antiphospholipid syndrome and asymptomatic carriers of antiphospholipid antibody: Prospective analysis of 404 individuals. *J Rheumatol*. 2004;31:1560–1567.
8. Lim W, Crowther MA, Eikelboom JW. Management of antiphospholipid antibody syndrome: A systematic review. *JAMA*. 2006;295:1050–7.
9. Miyakis S, Lockshin MD, Atsumi T, et al. International consensus statement on an update of the classification criteria for definite antiphospholipid syndrome (APS). *J Thromb Haemost*. 2006;4:295–306.
10. Gezer S. Antiphospholipid syndrome. *Dis Mon*. 2003;49:696–741.
11. Audrain MA, El-Kouri D, Hamidou MA, et al. Value of autoantibodies to beta(2)-glycoprotein 1 in the diagnosis of antiphospholipid syndrome. *Rheumatology (Oxford)*. 2002;41:550–553.
12. Espinosa G, Font J, Garcia-Pagan JC, et al. Budd-Chiari syndrome secondary to antiphospholipid syndrome: Clinical and immunologic characteristics of 43 patients. *Medicine (Baltimore)*. 2001;80:345–354.
13. Menon KV, Shah V, Kamath PS. The Budd-Chiari syndrome. *N Engl J Med*. 2004;350:578–585.
14. Finazzi G, Marchioli R, Brancaccio V, et al. A randomized clinical trial of high-intensity warfarin vs. conventional antithrombotic therapy for the prevention of recurrent thrombosis in patients with the antiphospholipid syndrome (WAPS). *J Thromb Haemost*. 2005;3:848–853.

15. Crowther MA, Ginsberg JS, Julian J, et al. A comparison of two intensities of warfarin for the prevention of recurrent thrombosis in patients with the antiphospholipid antibody syndrome. *N Engl J Med*. 2003;349:1133–1138.
16. Mueh JR, Herbst KD, Rapaport SI. Thrombosis in patients with the lupus anticoagulant. *Ann Intern Med*. 1980;92:156–159.
17. Purandare A, Godil MA, Prakash D, Parker R, Zerah M, Wilson TA. Spontaneous adrenal hemorrhage associated with transient antiphospholipid antibody in a child. *Clin Pediatr (Phila)*. 2001;40:347–350.
18. Gonzalez G, Gutierrez M, Ortiz M, Tellez R, Figueroa F, Jacobelli S. Association of primary antiphospholipid syndrome with primary adrenal insufficiency. *J Rheumatol*. 1996;23:1286–1287.
19. Arnason JA, Graziano FM. Adrenal insufficiency in the antiphospholipid antibody syndrome. *Semin Arthritis Rheum*. 1995;25:109–116.
20. Espinosa G, Santos E, Cervera R, et al. Adrenal involvement in the antiphospholipid syndrome: Clinical and immunologic characteristics of 86 patients. *Medicine (Baltimore)*. 2003;82:106–118.
21. Provenzale JM, Ortel TL, Nelson RC. Adrenal hemorrhage in patients with primary antiphospholipid syndrome: Imaging findings. *AJR Am J Roentgenol*. 1995;165:361–364.
22. Vella A, Nippoldt TB, Morris JC 3rd. Adrenal hemorrhage: A 25-year experience at the Mayo Clinic. *Mayo Clin Proc*. 2001;76:161–168.
23. Berneis K, Buitrago-Tellez C, Muller B, Keller U, Tsakiris DA. Antiphospholipid syndrome and endocrine damage: Why bilateral adrenal thrombosis? *Eur J Haematol*. 2003;71:299–302.
24. Boccarossa GN, Boccarossa SG. Reversible adrenal insufficiency after adrenal hemorrhage. *Ann Intern Med*. 1993;119:439–440.

CHAPTER **14**

CONSEQUENCES OF MISSED OPPORTUNITIES

JULIA C. DOMBROWSKI and HELEN KAO
Department of Medicine, University of California, San Francisco, California

NATASHA RENDA
School of Medicine, University of California, San Francisco, California

R. J. KOHLWES
Department of Medicine, University of California, San Francisco, California

A 58-year-old man was evaluated for 3 weeks of leg numbness and weakness. His symptoms began with numbness and tingling in the distal left leg that progressed to weakness that impaired his ability to walk. He had no history of trauma or incontinence but endorsed several months of back pain that worsened when lying flat. He had a history of type 2 diabetes mellitus, hepatitis C infection, hypertension, and posttraumatic stress disorder. He had a remote history of intravenous drug use and had quit tobacco 9 years earlier. Medications he was taking included hydrochlorothiazide, rosiglitazone, oxycodone/acetaminophen, baclofen, ibuprofen, and gabapentin.

Internists see this constellation of complaints frequently in an acute care setting. Finding a unifying diagnosis may be difficult initially, so thinking of the symptoms in series is helpful. The complaint of leg weakness and the pattern of numbness should be further elucidated. Is this true weakness, or is it a feeling of instability because of foot numbness? What is the pattern of the numbness? Peripheral neuropathy typically begins in a symmetric stocking pattern (involving the plantar surface of the feet), then progresses to a glove distribution (involving the hands from the fingers distally to the wrist proximally). Such a pattern in a patient with diabetes would be consistent with distal polyneuropathy, a mixed sensory and motor process. Other possible causes of peripheral neuropathy in this patient include HIV, B12 deficiency, and syphilis. These symptoms could be linked with the back pain if this were an intervertebral disk disease, a compression fracture, or a lytic lesion in the vertebrae with resulting nerve impingement or if it were an epidural spinal cord compression. The lack of bowel or bladder dysfunction speaks against a cauda equina syndrome but does not rule out more cephalad spinal pathology.

On neurological examination, I would concentrate on differentiating weakness from pain. I would attempt to determine whether the weakness was of central or peripheral nerve etiology. Helpful findings would include increased tone with upper motor lesions

Clinical Care Conundrums: Challenging Diagnoses in Hospital Medicine, First Edition.
Edited by James C. Pile, Thomas E. Baudendistel, and Brian J. Harte.

and flaccid tone with lower motor lesions, hyperreflexia with upper motor lesions and hyporeflexia with lower motor lesions, a Babinski sign, muscle atrophy or fasciculations, and gait. A rectal examination would also be helpful to assess for deficits in rectal tone, wink reflex, or saddle anesthesia.

All patients with low-back pain who have "alarm signs" of age more than 50 years, pain duration of more than 1 month, known cancer, lack of relief with conservative measures, or systemic "B" symptoms should undergo imaging of the spine. Although plain films may reveal bony abnormalities, computed tomography (CT) is better for evaluating osseous structures and magnetic resonance imaging (MRI) for evaluating pathology in patients suspected of having an infection or a malignancy. I would obtain imaging of the spine in this patient.

The patient was receiving care at an outside clinic for two liver lesions discovered on abdominal ultrasound 19 months prior to admission. CT showed that the lesions were 4.0 and 2.3 cm in diameter 17 months prior to admission and 5.0 and 3.0 cm in diameter 5 months prior to admission. No cirrhosis was appreciated on the ultrasound or CT. The patient was referred for CT-guided biopsy of the larger mass after the second CT, but he became anxious and left before the biopsy was obtained.

This piece of the history is ominous, as it increases the possibility of cancer in our differential. Metastatic disease could provide a unifying diagnosis, explaining the constellation of back pain, leg weakness, and liver lesions. Lung cancer commonly metastasizes to the liver and bone, so I would obtain a chest X-ray. Other possible types of cancer in this situation include cancer of the prostate, colon, or thyroid and melanoma. In this patient, who has hepatitis C, hepatocellular carcinoma (HCC) could be the primary etiology, although cirrhosis was not seen on CT and HCC metastasizes to the spine less commonly than do other primary cancers (e.g., lung, breast, prostate). Nonetheless, I would obtain an alpha-fetoprotein (AFP) level, which would confirm HCC in a patient with liver lesions if it was greater than 200 μg/L. Pancreatic cancer has been associated with both type 2 diabetes and liver lesions and could explain his abdominal pain.

There is no comment on the arterial-phase CT imaging of the liver lesions. Dual-phase CT scans examine the hepatic arterial and portal vein phases of contrast filling. Triple-phase CT scans also examine the portal vein influx phase. Both hemangiomas and hypervascular HCCs enhance on the arterial phase, as they derive their blood flow from the hepatic artery. Therefore, arterial-phase imaging can help distinguish vascular tumors that flush with contrast, such as hemangiomas, melanoma, and HCC, from less vascular tumors, such as pancreatic and colon cancer. Other liver lesions such as focal nodular hyperplasia and adenomas cannot be excluded in this situation because they also may enhance during the arterial phase and can grow over time, as this patient's repeat imaging documented. It seems unlikely that this patient has a liver abscess because he has a paucity of constitutional symptoms and no travel history. The liver lesions seen on initial imaging were larger than 1.0 cm, so I would have favored an earlier biopsy to obtain a tissue diagnosis.

The patient was afebrile, and all other vital signs were normal. He appeared well nourished and anicteric. There was no lymphadenopathy. Cardiac auscultation was regular without murmurs. The lungs were clear. The abdomen was without fluid wave or hepatosplenomegaly and was tender to palpation in the right

upper and lower quadrants. There was no midline tenderness to palpation of the spine.

Cranial nerves II–XII were intact. Lower extremity muscle tone could not be accurately assessed due to splinting from back pain. Strength was 3 of 5 in the left hip extensors and left knee flexors and extensors and 1 of 5 in the left hip flexors. He had no motor strength in the distal left lower extremity extensors. Bilateral upper extremity and right leg strength was normal. Sensation to light touch, temperature, and pain was decreased circumferentially below the xiphoid. The patient had hyperesthesia in a band around the thorax just above the xiphoid and paresthesia of the perineal area. Left patellar tendon reflexes were brisk, and left ankle jerk was absent, but other reflexes were normal. Toes were down-going bilaterally. The anal wink was absent, and rectal tone was decreased. Results of the cerebellar exam were normal. Gait could not be assessed.

The results of the exam are notable for not showing the stigmata of end-stage liver disease. The results of the neurological exam are concerning, with decreased sensation at approximately the T7 level that is almost certainly a result of epidural compression of the spinal cord. Hematogenous metastasis to the vertebrae from one of the tumors mentioned above, with spread into the thecal sac, is the most likely cause. An epidural abscess is possible because the patient has diabetes and a history of injection drug use.

The thoracic spine is involved in 60% of spinal cord metastases. This patient's left-sided distal leg weakness is consistent with having corticospinal tract compression and indicates thoracic spine involvement. Flaccid paralysis is classically found in lower motor neuron weakness but is also seen in the early stages of upper motor neuron pathology. Lesions found above the cauda equina often spare the perineal area, but low thoracic lesions involving the conus medullaris (from T10 to L1) could explain both his loss of anal wink and his decreased rectal tone.

This patient's presentation is unfortunately classic for epidural spinal cord compression. Because the onset of compression is insidious, the diagnosis is often delayed, even in patients with known cancer. Urgent imaging is imperative to evaluate this possibility, as having any meaningful chance of recovery of function depends on rapid relief of the spinal cord compression. I would obtain an emergent MRI of the thoracic and lumbosacral spine.

Laboratory studies showed the following: hemoglobin, 13.1 g/dL; mean corpuscular volume, 80 μm^3; platelet count, 149,000/L; creatinine, 1.9 mg/dL; aspartate aminotransferase, 66 U/L (5–35 U/L); alanine aminotransferase, 66 U/L (7–56 U/L); alkaline phosphatase, 87 U/L (40–125 U/L); total bilirubin, 1.3 mg/dL; prostate-specific antigen (PSA), 1.6 μg/dL; and AFP, 10.3 μg/L. White blood cell count, sodium, glucose, calcium, and albumin levels, and prothrombin and partial-thromboplastin times were within normal ranges.

His liver function tests likely reflect chronic hepatitis C infection. His renal insufficiency could be a result of hypertension, diabetes, or dehydration given that he has been bedbound.

Most intriguing are the normal PSA level and only slightly elevated AFP level. PSA is useful for detecting recurrence of prostate cancer or following response of therapy, but the utility of PSA as a screening tool remains controversial in part because of its low specificity. Prostate cancer is the most commonly diagnosed cancer among men and cannot be ruled out by a normal PSA. In a patient with hepatitis C, cirrhosis (which we have not conclusively diagnosed), and a radiologically suspicious liver lesion, an

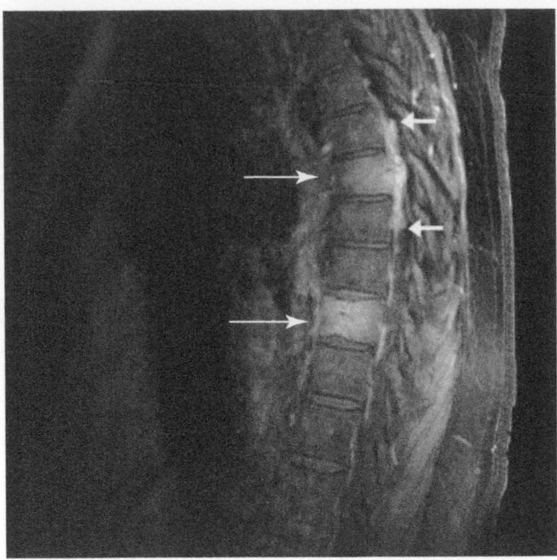

FIGURE 14.1 T2-weighted thoracic MRI with gadolinium showing complete marrow replacement of the T7 and T10 vertebral bodies (arrows on left). Invasion of the posterior cortex with epidural extension of enhancing soft tissue from T6 to T8 (right arrows) results in cord compression at the T7 level.

AFP > 200 μg/L would be diagnostic of HCC. In this case, however, mildly elevated AFP does not help us to either diagnose or exclude HCC.

The chest X-ray showed no abnormalities. MRI of the spine revealed lytic lesions in the T7–T10 vertebral bodies with spinal cord compression at the T7 level (Fig. 14.1).

A repeat CT scan of the abdomen showed a coarse, nodular liver with two heterogeneous early-enhancing masses (4.7 × 4.2 and 3.4 × 2.4 cm in diameter) with surrounding satellite lesions (Fig. 14.2).

The enhancement pattern on dual-phase liver protocol CT was not characteristic of HCC. The left portal vein was not visualized. Splenomegaly and esophageal varices were observed. The adrenal glands showed bilateral, heterogeneous enhancing masses. The epiphrenic, retroperitoneal, and periportal lymph nodes were enlarged. Lytic lesions were seen in the sacrum, left iliac wing, and T7–T10 vertebral bodies.

Intravenous high-dose steroids were started. The neurosurgery team advised that no surgical interventions were appropriate because of the patient's poor functional status and the extent of his disease.

It is unfortunate that no neurosurgical interventions could help this patient, especially because we are not yet sure of the final diagnosis. Standard indications for neurosurgical decompression include compression from bone fragments, spinal instability requiring fixation, and lack of response to radiation therapy. Patients must also be able to tolerate surgery. Although evidence supports the use of corticosteroids in reducing edema, inflammation, and neurological deficits in malignant spinal cord compression, there is no consensus on what the optimal dose is. Doses of 16–100 mg of dexamethasone per day appear to be beneficial, as long as higher doses are rapidly tapered to avoid toxic effects. High-dose steroids minimize the initial edema but are unlikely to change the long-term outcome of patients who are nonambulatory on arrival.

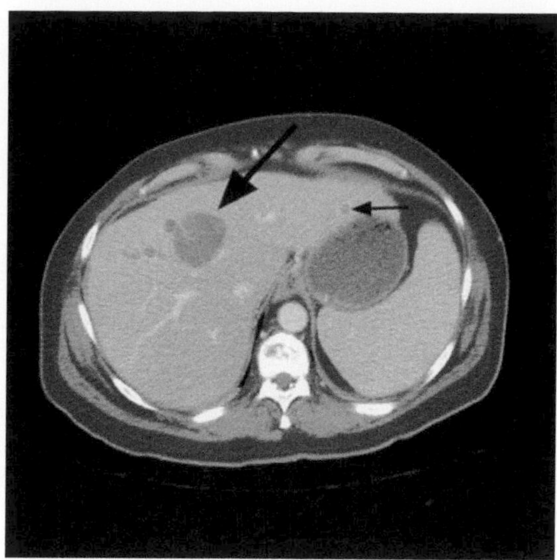

FIGURE 14.2 Contrast-enhanced CT of the abdomen using dual-phase liver protocol during the arterial phase showing the largest (4.7 × 4.2 cm) of two dominant heterogeneously enhancing masses in the liver near the junction of the right and left lobes (large arrow). There are also multiple, low-attenuation, satellite lesions surrounding the dominant lesion and a ring-enhancing lesion (8 mm) (small arrow) in segment 2 of the liver.

The CT scan does not help us distinguish between metastatic cancer and primary HCC. Adrenal metastases are very uncommon in HCC. Lung cancer, however, metastasizes to the liver, adrenal glands, and spine, even without significant pulmonary symptoms. HCC may be seen on CT as a solitary mass, a dominant mass with surrounding satellite lesions, multifocal lesions, or a diffusely infiltrating tumor. This diagnosis now seems more likely given the finding of cirrhosis, which increases the risk of HCC in individuals with hepatitis C infection.

We need to obtain tissue for diagnosis and prognosis and to guide therapy. I would consult with my radiology and gastroenterology colleagues about the best location to perform biopsy on, but a bone biopsy should be avoided because the pathologic yield is lower.

The radiology and gastroenterology consultants recommended adrenal biopsy because there was easier posterior access for tissue. A liver biopsy was avoided because of the risk of bleeding with hypervascular masses. Fine-needle aspiration of the mass in the right adrenal gland was performed. The pathology demonstrated bile production and hexagonal arrangement of cells with endothelial cuffing consistent with HCC. The oncology staff was consulted about palliative chemotherapy options. The patient began radiation therapy directed at the T7 lesion compressing the spinal cord. He regained minimal movement of his foot. After discussing treatment options with the oncology staff, the patient declined chemotherapy and was transitioned to hospice, where he died 3 weeks later.

COMMENTARY

HCC is the third-leading cause of cancer death and the fifth-leading cause of cancer worldwide. It causes nearly 1 million deaths annually, and unlike many other cancers, its incidence and mortality rate are rising. Most cases of HCC in Africa and Asia are a result of chronic hepatitis B infection, but in the United States, HCC is primarily attributable to hepatitis C infection.[1] The annual incidence of HCC in the US population, about 4 cases per 100,000 people,[2] is rising because of the increased prevalence of hepatitis C infection. Other causes of HCC, such as alcoholic liver disease, hepatitis B infection, and hemochromatosis, have remained stable and have not contributed as significantly to the rising incidence of HCC. For the individual patient, hepatitis C infection conveys a 20-fold increase in the risk for HCC (2%–8% risk per year).[1] Eighty percent of cases of HCC develop in patients with cirrhosis.[3] Unlike patients with hepatitis B infection, persons chronically infected with hepatitis C rarely develop HCC unless they have cirrhosis.

The American Association for the Study of Liver Diseases (AASLD) recommends that hepatitis-B-infected individuals at high risk for HCC (e.g., men older than 40 years and persons with cirrhosis or a family history of HCC) and hepatitis-C-infected individuals with cirrhosis[4] be periodically screened for HCC with AFP and ultrasonography (every 6 months to approximate the doubling time of the tumor[5]). Using the most commonly reported cutoff for a positive test result for HCC (AFP level > 20 μg/L) resulted in the following test characteristics: sensitivity, 41%–65%; specificity, 80%–94%; positive likelihood ratio, 3.1–6.8; and negative likelihood ratio, 0.4–0.6.[6] AFP alone is therefore a poor screening test for HCC, and as shown in this case, AFP levels can be normal or only minimally elevated in the setting of diffusely metastatic disease. Ultrasonography alone is only 35%–87% sensitive in detecting HCC,[7–9] but the combination of AFP and ultrasonography identified 100% of HCC cases in one small case series.[10]

For the patient in this case, the optimal clinical pathway would have been to transition from screening to diagnostic measures in a timely manner. Consensus guidelines from the European Association for the Study of the Liver (EASL) in 2001 recommend biopsy of all focal liver lesions that are between 1 and 2 cm.[11] The AASLD recommends that focal liver lesions between 1 and 2 cm found on ultrasound in cirrhotic livers be followed by two dynamic studies: CT, MRI, or contrast ultrasound. If two separate studies reveal typical characteristics of HCC, the lesion should be treated as HCC, and if not typical, the lesion should be biopsied.[4] Although no studies were available to support the recommendations, both the EASL and AASLD advise that lesions of size greater than 2 cm with demonstrated vascularity on both ultrasonography and CT can be diagnosed as HCC without biopsy and that lesions smaller than 1 cm be monitored.[4,11]

HCC can metastasize to almost anywhere in the body by hematologic or lymphatic spread or by direct extension. The most common site for metastases of HCC is the lung. Metastases to the lung arise primarily from arterial emboli and therefore are most common in the lower lobes, where there is greater perfusion.[12] The second most common site is the intra-abdominal lymph nodes. The axial skeleton is the third most common site of metastases and, as in this case, primarily involves the spine.[13] Other sites of metastases include the peritoneum, the inferior vena cava and right atrium by direct extension, and, less commonly, the gallbladder and spleen. Autopsy studies of patients with HCC found that 8% had metastases to the adrenal glands, as did this patient.[13] Metastasis to the central nervous system is rare.

Key Points

1. Patients infected with hepatitis C who are found to have suspicious hepatic lesions should be aggressively evaluated for HCC.
2. Using an AFP level <20 μg/L as a screening test is not helpful because this level can be seen even with widely metastatic disease.

3. In patients with chronic hepatitis C virus infection, HCC rarely occurs unless cirrhosis is present.

REFERENCES

1. Sherman MS. Hepatocellular carcinoma: Epidemiology, risk factors, and screening. *Semin Liver Dis*. 2005;25:143–154.
2. American Cancer Society. Cancer Facts and Figures 2005. Atlanta, GA: American Cancer Society, 2005. Available at: http://www.cancer.org/docroot/STT/stt_0.asp. Accessed October 17, 2005.
3. Llovet JM, Burroughs A, Bruix J. Hepatocellular carcinoma. *Lancet*. 2003;362:1907–1917.
4. Bruix J, Sherman M. Management of hepatocellular carcinoma. AASLD Practice Guideline. *Hepatology*. 2005;42:1208–1236.
5. Sheu JC, Sung JL, Chen DS, et al. Growth rate of asymptomatic hepatocellular carcinoma and its clinical implications. *Gastroenterology*. 1985;89:259–266.
6. Gupta S, Bent S, Kohlwes J. Test characteristics of alpha-fetoprotein for detecting hepatocellular carcinoma in patients with hepatitis C. *Ann Intern Med*. 2003;139:46–50.
7. Larcos G, Sorokopud H, Berry G, Farrell GC. Sonographic screening for hepatocellular carcinoma in patients with chronic hepatitis or cirrhosis: An evaluation. *Am J Roentgenol*. 1998;171:433–435.
8. Dodd GD 3rd, Miller WJ, Baron RL, Skolnick ML, Campbell WL. Detection of malignant tumors in end-stage cirrhotic livers: Efficacy of sonography as a screening technique. *Am J Roentgenol*. 1992;159:727–733.
9. Takayasu K, Moriyama N, Muramatsu Y, et al. The diagnosis of small hepatocellular carcinomas: Efficacy of various imaging procedures in 100 patients. *Am J Roentgenol*. 1990;155:49–54.
10. Izzo F, Cremona F, Ruffolo F, Palaia R, Parisi V, Curley SA. Outcome of 67 patients with hepatocellular cancer detected during screening of 1125 patients with chronic hepatitis. *Ann Surg*. 1998;277:513–518.
11. Bruix J, Sherman M, Llovet JM, et al. EASL Panel of Experts on HCC. Clinical management of hepatocellular carcinoma. Conclusions of the Barcelona-2000 EASL conference. European Association for the Study of the Liver. *J Hepatol*. 2001;35:421–430.
12. Hong SS, Kim TK, Sung K-B, et al. Extrahepatic spread of hepatocellular carcinoma: A pictorial review. *Eur Radiol*. 2003;13:874–882.
13. Katyal S, Oliver JH III, Peterson MS, Ferris JV, Carr BS, Baron RL. Extrahepatic metastases of hepatocellular carcinoma. *Radiology*. 2000;216:698–703.

CHAPTER 15

IN SIGHT BUT OUT OF MIND

LETIZIA ATTALA
University of Florence Medical School, Florence, Italy

ADAM TREMBLAY
Ann Arbor Veterans Affairs Medical Center, University of Michigan, Ann Arbor, Michigan

GIAMPAOLO CORTI
University of Florence Medical School, Florence, Italy

SANJAY SAINT
Department of Internal Medicine, University of Michigan, Ann Arbor, Michigan; Ann Arbor VA Health Services Research and Development Field Program, Ann Arbor, Michigan; Patient Safety Enhancement Program, University of Michigan Health System, Ann Arbor, Michigan; Tuscan-American Safety, Collaborative, Florence, Italy

ALESSANDRO BARTOLONI
University of Florence Medical School, Florence, Italy; Tuscan-American Safety Collaborative, Florence, Italy

A 44-year-old woman was admitted to an Italian hospital with fever and chills that had started approximately 1 week earlier. A few days after onset of fever, she had noticed a red, nonpruritic, confluent, maculopapular rash that began on her face and descended to her body. She also complained of red eyes, photophobia, dyspnea, and watery diarrhea. She denied nausea, vomiting, headache, or neck stiffness. She had seen her primary care physician who had concomitantly prescribed amoxicillin, levofloxacin, and betamethasone. She took the medications for several days without symptomatic improvement.

The salient features of this acute illness include the maculopapular rash, fever, and red eyes with photophobia. The differential diagnosis includes infections, rheumatologic disorders, toxin exposure, and, less likely, hematologic malignancies. In the initial assessment, it is crucial to rule out any life-threatening etiologies of fever and rash, such as septicemia from *Neisseria meningitidis*, bacterial endocarditis, toxic shock syndrome, typhoid fever, and rickettsial diseases. A number of critical components of the history would help narrow the diagnostic considerations, including any history of recent travel, animal or occupational exposure, sexual or medication history, and risk factors for immunosuppression.

The empiric use of antibiotics is indicated when a patient presents with symptoms that suggest life-threatening illness. For nonemergent conditions, empiric antibiotics may

Clinical Care Conundrums: Challenging Diagnoses in Hospital Medicine, First Edition.
Edited by James C. Pile, Thomas E. Baudendistel, and Brian J. Harte.

be appropriate when a classic pattern for a given diagnosis is present. In this patient, however, the initial presentation neither appears to be life-threatening nor is it easily recognizable as a specific or classic diagnosis. Thus, I would not start antibiotics, because doing so may further disguise the diagnosis by interfering with culture results or it complicate the case by causing an adverse effect such as fever or rash.

One week before the onset of fever, she went to the emergency department because of pain in both lower quadrants of her abdomen. The physician removed her intrauterine device (IUD), which appeared to be partially expelled. The patient returned the next day to the emergency department because of severe metrorrhagia.

Complications of IUDs include pelvic inflammatory disease, perforated uterus, myometrial abscess, partial or complete spontaneous abortion, and ectopic pregnancy. Toxic shock syndrome, pelvic inflammatory disease, and retained products from a partial spontaneous abortion can all lead to significant systemic disease and vaginal bleeding.

Her past medical history was unremarkable except for an episode of bacterial meningitis 20 years before. She lived in Florence, Italy, where she worked as a school teacher and had not traveled outside of Italy in the last year. She was married, with two children, and denied high-risk sexual behavior. She did not own any animals.

The patient's lack of travel, high-risk sexual behavior, or animal exposure does not help alter the differential diagnosis. The prior history of bacterial meningitis raises the question of an immunodeficiency syndrome. At this point, I remain concerned about toxic shock syndrome.

The patient's temperature was 38.2°C; blood pressure, 110/60 mm Hg; respiratory rate, 28 breaths per minute; and heart rate, 108 beats per minute. She was alert and oriented but appeared moderately ill. Her conjunctivae were hyperemic without any drainage, and her oropharynx was erythematous. Lung examination revealed diminished breath sounds in the lower right lung field and crackles bilaterally. Abdominal exam demonstrated mild hepatomegaly, but not splenomegaly. Skin exam showed an erythematous, confluent, maculopapular rash involving her face, torso, back, and extremities; no cutaneous abscesses were noted. Neurological and gynecological exams were both normal, as was the rectal examination.

Her vital signs suggest a progressive illness and possible sepsis. The conjunctival hyperemia could represent several pathologic findings including uveitis with ciliary flush, conjunctival hemorrhage, or hyperemia due to systemic illness. The pulmonary findings could be attributed to pulmonary edema, pneumonia, alveolar hemorrhage, or acute respiratory distress syndrome (ARDS) as a complication of sepsis and systemic inflammation. The hepatomegaly, while nonspecific, may be due to an inflammatory reaction to a systemic illness. If so, I would expect liver tests to be elevated, as this can occur in a number of parasitic (e.g., toxoplasmosis) and viral (e.g., chickenpox, infectious mononucleosis, cytomegalovirus) infections. The lack of concurrent splenomegaly makes lymphoma or other hematologic malignancies less likely. Given the patient's constellation of symptoms, the progressive nature of her illness, and the multiple organs involved, I continue to be most concerned about immediately life-threatening diseases. Toxic shock syndrome secondary to staphylococcal infection can present with many of these signs and symptoms including conjunctival hyperemia, diffuse maculopapular erythema, pharyngitis and sepsis leading to pulmonary edema, pleural effusions, and ARDS. Another possibility is leptospirosis, which can be associated with pharyngitis, hepatomegaly, diffuse rash, low-grade fever, and frequently has conjunctival hyperemia. Moreover, leptospirosis has a markedly variable course and pulmonary hemorrhage and

ARDS can occur in severe cases. However, the lack of clear exposure to an environmental source such as contaminated water or soil or animal tissue reduces my enthusiasm for it.

Routine laboratory studies demonstrated the following: white blood cell count, 5210/mm^3 (82% neutrophils, 10% lymphocytes, 7% monocytes, and 1% eosinophils); hematocrit, 36.3%; platelet count, 135,000/mm^3; erythrocyte sedimentation rate, 49 mm/hour; fibrinogen, 591 mg/dL (normal range, 200–450 mg/dL); and C-reactive protein, 53 mg/L (normal range, $<$9 mg/L). Serum electrolyte levels were normal. Liver tests demonstrated the following: aspartate aminotransferase, 75 U/L; alanine aminotransferase, 135 U/L; total bilirubin was within normal limits; and gamma glutamyltransferase, 86 U/L (normal range, 10–40 U/L). The urea nitrogen and the creatinine were both normal. The creatine phosphokinase was 381 U/L. Urinalysis was normal. An arterial blood gas, obtained while the patient was breathing room air, revealed an oxygen saturation of 87%, pH of 7.45, pCO_2 of 38 mm Hg, pO_2 of 54 mm Hg, and bicarbonate concentration of 27 mmol/L.

Her electrocardiogram was normal except for sinus tachycardia. Chest film revealed a right-sided pleural effusion without evidence of parenchymal abnormalities (Fig. 15.1).

Despite the systemic illness, fever, and markedly abnormal inflammatory markers, the white blood cell count remains normal with a slight leftward shift. The most alarming finding is hypoxemia seen on the arterial blood gas. My leading diagnoses for this multisystemic febrile illness with a rash and hypoxia continue to be primarily infectious etiologies, including toxic shock syndrome with *Staphylococcus* species, leptospirosis, acute cytomegalovirus, and mycobacterial infections. Further diagnostic tests need to be performed, but I would begin empiric antibiotics after appropriate cultures have been obtained. Rheumatologic etiologies such as systemic lupus erythematosus (SLE) and sarcoidosis seem less likely. SLE can present with a systemic illness, fever, and rash, but hepatitis, hepatomegaly, and hyperemic conjunctivae are less common.

At the time of hospital admission, blood cultures were obtained before azithromycin, meropenem, and vancomycin were initiated for presumed toxic shock

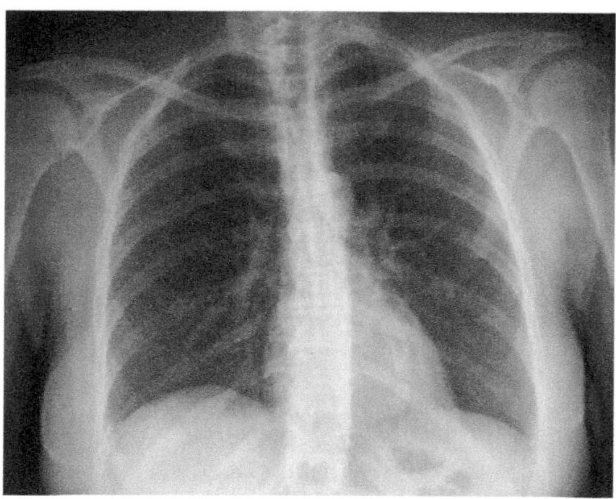

FIGURE 15.1 Posterior-anterior chest film, revealing small right pleural effusion.

syndrome. Transvaginal and abdominal ultrasound studies revealed no abnormalities. She remained febrile, but blood cultures returned negative. The results of the following investigations were also negative: (i) immunoglobulin M (IgM) antibodies against *Chlamydophila pneumoniae*, cytomegalovirus, Epstein–Barr virus, *Legionella pneumophila*, parvovirus B19, rubella virus, *Coxiella burnetii*, *Mycoplasma pneumoniae*, *Chlamydophila psittaci*, adenovirus, and coxsackieviruses; (ii) antibodies against human immunodeficiency virus (HIV) 1 and 2; and (iii) tests for hepatitis B (HB surface antigen [HbsAg] and HB core antibody [HbcAb] IgM) and C (HCV-Ab) viruses.

The lack of IgM antibodies for the infections listed markedly reduces their likelihood but does not exclude them. For example, given that the duration of symptoms is nearly 2 weeks at this point, it is possible that IgM has already decreased and IgG titers are now present. The lack of positive cultures does not exclude toxic shock syndrome, since in many severe cases, the cultures remain negative. Thus, I remain concerned about toxic shock syndrome and would continue broad-spectrum antibiotics.

After further investigating possible ill contacts to which the patient could have been exposed, it emerged that in the previous weeks, there had been a case of measles in the kindergarten where she was working. The patient did not recall her vaccination history.

The recent exposure raises the risk of measles significantly, especially if she was not immunized as a child.

Measles typically has an incubation period of 10–14 days, thus the prior exposure would fit the time course for the onset of this patient's symptoms. In retrospect, many of this patient's symptoms are classic for measles, including the maculopapular rash that begins on the face and extends downward, the conjunctival hyperemia, the persistent low-grade fever, and the lack of clinical response to antibiotics.

In adults, measles can be complicated by inflammation in multiple organs resulting in myocarditis, pericarditis, hepatitis, encephalitis, and pneumonia. Thus, elevated transaminases would be consistent with the diagnosis as would a normal abdominal ultrasound. The pneumonia may be due to the measles infection itself or the coexisting viral or bacterial infections. The findings of a mild thrombocytopenia and a low normal leukocyte count can also be seen in measles infection. The diagnosis of measles is based on clinical presentation and by serologic confirmation: IgM antibodies are detectable within 1 or 2 days after the appearance of the rash, whereas the IgG titer rises significantly after 10 days.

I would continue the broad-spectrum antibiotics until measles serologies could be confirmed. If the measles serologies are negative, I would continue the evaluation. If the serologies are positive, however, I would continue supportive care and review her pulmonary status to make sure she does not have a secondary bacterial infection. I strongly suspect that she has measles that is complicated by pneumonia and hepatitis.

The IgM antibody against measles virus returned positive and the patient was diagnosed with measles. By hospital day 5, her fever disappeared, her dyspnea resolved, and her rash had receded. Her oxygen saturation was 97% at the time of discharge.

COMMENTARY

Measles is a highly contagious, acute-onset, exanthematous disease that affects the respiratory tract and mucous membranes. Measles is clinically characterized by a prodromal stage of cough, conjunctivitis, coryza and high fever, typically lasting between 2 and 4 days.[1,2] The pathognomonic finding on the oral mucosa (Koplik spots) is usually followed by a generalized rash. The characteristic rash of measles is erythematous, nonpruritic, and maculopapular beginning at the hairline and behind the ears, and then spreads down the trunk and limbs and may include the palms and soles.[1,2] Often the patient has diarrhea, vomiting, lymphadenopathy, and splenomegaly; however, the clinical presentation can vary.[1,2] In partially immunized patients, symptoms are often atypical, whereas severe cases are characteristically seen in adults with the most frequent complication being pneumonia. About 3% of young adults with measles have viral pneumonia that requires hospitalization.[2–4] Adults are much more likely than children to develop hepatitis, bronchospasm, and bacterial superinfection.[2,3,5]

The introduction of the measles vaccine initially led to a dramatic decrease in the incidence of measles. However, lack of adherence to vaccination campaigns among some families has been followed by small epidemics. Childhood vaccination rates against measles have recently been reported as 88% in Italy, and even higher—over 90%—in Tuscany. However, Italy has faced an upsurge of measles since September 2007, with almost 60% of cases occurring in the 15- to 44-year-old age group.[6]

Classic presentations of common diseases are easily recognized, but in those cases in which the clinical presentation of uncommon illnesses—such as measles in adults—is atypical, the epidemiological data and the clinical history play key roles. In this patient, both the discussant and clinical team focused on the most alarming potential diagnosis: toxic shock syndrome related to the use of the IUD. While appropriate, there were historical clues that this patient had measles that were not specifically sought—the immunization status and the workplace (school) exposure.

This case highlights two important aspects of making a difficult clinical diagnosis. First, the patient did not recall her immunization history, and the clinical team did not clarify it, and thus potential childhood illnesses such as measles and rubella did not remain on the differential diagnosis. Assuming that a patient has had the appropriate vaccinations is done at the clinician's—and the patient's—peril. Second, many diseases that commonly afflict children can also occur in adult patients, albeit less frequently. Had this patient been a 5-year-old child with the same symptoms, the diagnosis would likely have been made with alacrity. However, maculopapular rashes that begin on the face and spread to the body are quite uncommon in adult medicine. For both the discussant and the clinical team, the rash was clearly in sight but the correct diagnosis was out of mind given the rarity of this infection in adults. Fortunately, however, once it became clear that the patient was unlikely to have toxic shock syndrome, the epidemiological detail initially left behind became the sentinel clue necessary to solve the case.

Key Points

1. After nearly vanishing in the developed world, measles has shown sporadic signs of resurgence in recent years. The disease needs to be considered in patients presenting with a febrile illness accompanied by an exanthem that begins on the head and spreads inferiorly, especially when accompanied by cough, rhinorrhea, and conjunctival changes.
2. Measles tends to cause relatively severe illness and frequent complications in adults, the most common of which is pneumonia.

REFERENCES

1. Gershon AA. Measles virus (rubeola). In: Mandell GL, Bennett JE, Dolin R, eds. *Mandell, Douglas and Bennett's Principles and Practice of Infectious Diseases*. 6th ed. Philadelphia, PA: Elsevier Churchill Livingstone; 2005:2031–2038.
2. Perry RT, Halsey NA. The clinical significance of measles: A review. *J Infect Dis*. 2004;189(Suppl 1): S4–S16.
3. Asaria P, MacMahon E. Measles in the United Kingdom: Can we eradicate it by 2010? *Br Med J*. 2006;333:890–895.
4. Ito I, Ishida T, Hashimoto T, Arita M, Osawa M, Tsukayama C. Familial cases of severe measles pneumonia. *Intern Med*. 2000;39:670–674.
5. Takebayashi K, Aso Y, Wakabayashi S, et al. Measles encephalitis and acute pancreatitis in a young adult. *Am J Med Sci*. 2004;327:299–303.
6. Filia A, De Crescenzo M, Seyler T, et al. Measles resurges in Italy: Preliminary data from September 2007 to May 2008. *Euro Surveill*. 2008;13(29):pii:18928.

CHAPTER **16**

A CHANGE OF HEART

JONATHAN P. PICCINI and ADRIAN F. HERNANDEZ
Division of Cardiovascular Medicine, Duke Clinical Research Institute, Duke University Medical Center, Duke University, Durham, North Carolina

LOUIS R. DIBERNARDO
Department of Pathology, Duke University Medical Center, Duke University, Durham, North Carolina

JOSEPH G. ROGERS
Division of Cardiovascular Medicine, Duke Clinical Research Institute, Duke University Medical Center, Duke University, Durham, North Carolina

GURPREET DHALIWAL
Department of Medicine, University of California, San Francisco, California; Medical Service, San Francisco VA Medical Center, San Francisco, California

A 29-year-old man developed palpitations and dyspnea while loading boxes into a truck. In the emergency department, telemetry demonstrated a wide-complex tachycardia at a rate of 204 beats per minute. The patient spontaneously cardioverted to sinus rhythm (Fig. 16.1).

Wide-complex tachycardia is usually explained by a supraventricular tachycardia with aberrant ventricular conduction or a ventricular tachycardia. Although algorithms exist to guide the clinician in sorting through those etiologies, often the knowledge of underlying structural cardiac disease is most informative. In patients with a history of myocardial infarction, greater than 95% of wide-complex tachycardia is ventricular tachycardia. Ventricular ectopy, T-wave inversion or flattening, and poor R-wave progression are suggestive of a cardiomyopathy, either acute or chronic. A pressing concern, especially with the Q waves and concave ST morphology in V1 and V2, would be coronary ischemia. His age makes this less likely, but an aberrant coronary circulation or drug use could account for it.

Over the past 2 years, the patient had several episodes of sustained palpitations, which terminated after several minutes. Previously, the patient exercised frequently, including playing rugby in college. However, over the past year, he experienced difficulty climbing stairs due to shortness of breath, which he attributed to deconditioning and smoking. He had no significant medical history, was not taking any medications, and did not use recreational stimulants. He drank alcohol occasionally. He had no risk factors for the human immunodeficiency virus (HIV). Both of the patient's parents were alive and well. There was no family history of sudden cardiac death.

Clinical Care Conundrums: Challenging Diagnoses in Hospital Medicine, First Edition.
Edited by James C. Pile, Thomas E. Baudendistel, and Brian J. Harte.

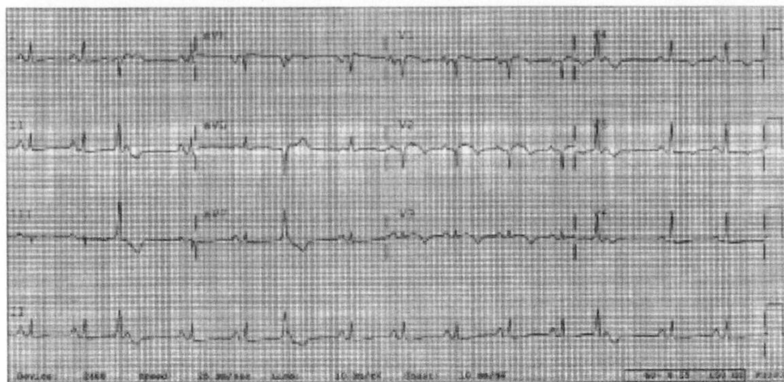

FIGURE 16.1 Twelve-lead electrocardiogram demonstrating biatrial abnormalities, premature ventricular complexes, precordial ST-segment abnormalities, and precordial T-wave inversion in leads V1 through V5. Noted is the presence of a low-amplitude signal in the early ST-segment in leads V1 and V2, which could represent an epsilon wave.

The duration of symptoms suggests that this is a chronic cardiomyopathy rather than acute myocarditis or acute ischemia, acknowledging that either one could be superimposed. The absence of family history lowers the likelihood of heritable causes of arrhythmia that may accompany a structurally normal (e.g., long QT syndrome) or abnormal (e.g., hypertrophic cardiomyopathy) heart, although penetrance can be variable. Most cases of cardiomyopathy in young patients are probably idiopathic, but etiologies that diverge from the usual suspects of coronary artery disease, hypertension, and valvular disease, which affect older population, include antecedent viral myocarditis, substance abuse, HIV, and infiltrative disorders such as sarcoidosis.

The patient's pulse was 92 beats per minute and regular and the blood pressure was 96/52 mm Hg. The jugular venous pressure was elevated with prominent v waves, the point of maximal impulse was diffuse, there were no extra heart sounds or murmurs, and an enlarged liver was detected. An echocardiogram demonstrated left ventricular dysfunction with an ejection fraction of 30%, severe enlargement of the right atrium and right ventricle, and moderate tricuspid regurgitation. Cardiac catheterization revealed normal coronary arteries without evidence of pulmonary hypertension or intracardiac shunt.

The physical examination and echocardiographic findings of right-sided failure are unusual given the absence of pulmonary hypertension or intracardiac shunt and could prompt repeat of the hemodynamic measurements and/or investigations for pulmonary disease that may account for right-sided pressure overload (in addition to that caused by left ventricular failure). An alternative explanation would be a cardiomyopathic process that preferentially involves the right side of the heart, such as arrhythmogenic right ventricular dysplasia (ARVD), but that would not satisfactorily explain the significant decline in left ventricular function. An acute right ventricular infarction could cause his acute symptoms and his examination and echocardiographic findings, but not the underlying chronic illness. It is common to see patients with long-standing biventricular failure who present with prominent signs of right-sided failure (elevated neck veins, hepatomegaly, and edema) but limited or no signs of left-sided failure (rales) to match their degree of volume overload or dyspnea.

Cardiac magnetic resonance imaging (MRI) revealed a dilated right ventricle with extensive hyperenhancement, a right ventricular ejection fraction of 9%, and

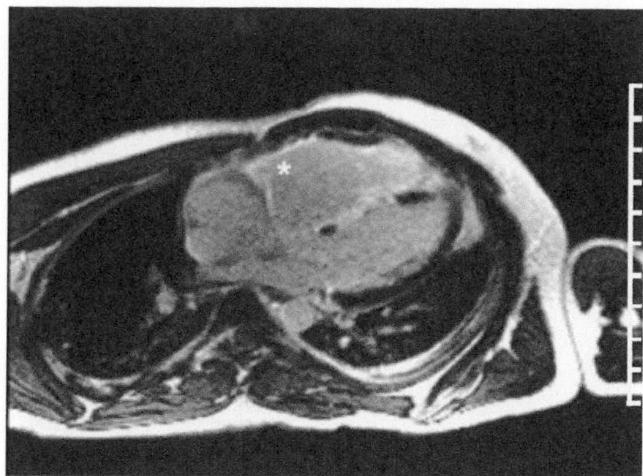

FIGURE 16.2 Cardiac magnetic resonance imaging demonstrated severe right atrial and right ventricular enlargement (asterisk denotes right ventricle), severe right ventricular dysfunction, and moderate left ventricular dysfunction. As shown here, gadolinium administration revealed extensive transmural right ventricular hyperenhancement. Delayed enhancement was also noted in the septum and basal portions of the left ventricle.

moderate left ventricular dysfunction (Fig. 16.2). Electrophysiology testing induced both nonsustained polymorphic and monomorphic ventricular tachycardia. Late potentials were detected on a signal-averaged electrocardiogram. A single-chamber cardioverter defibrillator was implanted and the patient was discharged on carvedilol, lisinopril, and spironolactone. The HIV-1 antibody test was negative, and the thyroid-stimulating hormone concentration was within normal limits.

Assuming that accurate evaluation of the pulmonary circulation has been undertaken to exclude pulmonary hypertension, the enlarged and hyperenhanced right ventricle on MRI suggests a process that preferentially infiltrates the right ventricular myocardium and may secondarily affect the left ventricle either by further infiltration or as a consequence of altered mechanics from the highly dysfunctional right ventricle. ARVD affects the right ventricle, but it is possible that another infiltrative cardiomyopathy, such as sarcoid or an antecedent viral infection, could be restricted in its distribution. Late potentials identified on signal-averaged electrocardiograms indicate areas of abnormal conduction that may serve as substrate for reentrant ventricular arrhythmias. They are, however, nonspecific, as they are seen in a variety of myocardial diseases.

The patient continued to have progressive dyspnea and was readmitted after receiving an appropriate implantable cardioverter defibrillator shock for ventricular tachycardia. Recurrent slow ventricular tachycardia (Fig. 16.3) was treated with supplemental beta-blockade and amiodarone (10 g total). Repeat echocardiography demonstrated severe left ventricular dysfunction with an ejection fraction of less than 15%. There were no recurrences of ventricular arrhythmias and the patient was discharged and referred for cardiac transplant evaluation for ARVD.

This degree of left ventricular dysfunction is unlikely to be accounted for by altered mechanics and interactions from a failing right ventricle alone and frames this as a biventricular cardiomyopathy, which has an extensive differential diagnosis.

On routine laboratory testing 6 months later, a serum aspartate aminotransferase of 79 U/L and a serum alanine aminotransferase of 118 U/L were found. Bilirubin, albumin, and alkaline phosphatase were normal. The transaminase levels had been normal on initial evaluation. The patient reported that his two paternal

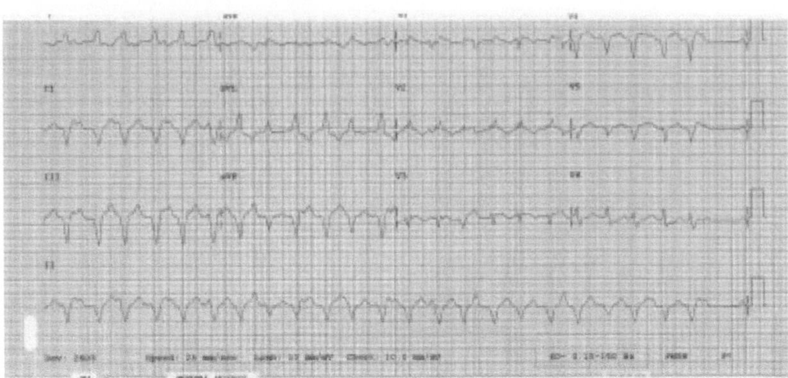

FIGURE 16.3 Twelve-lead electrocardiogram obtained after hospitalization for an implantable cardioverter defibrillator shock. Note the presence of wide-complex tachycardia and atrioventricular dissociation consistent with ventricular tachycardia. Terminal S waves in leads I, V6, and an RSR pattern in V1 suggest a right bundle branch-like morphology, and thus left ventricular origin.

uncles had end-stage nonalcoholic cirrhosis. Transjugular liver biopsy was consistent with mild lobular hepatitis with mild portal fibrosis with a few lobular collections of mononuclear cells. There was no evidence of iron overload. The hepatic venogram and transhepatic pressure gradient (2 mm Hg) were normal.

The elevated transaminase levels could be due to amiodarone-associated hepatotoxicity, hepatic congestion, or a primary liver disease. It is important to consider combined cardiohepatic syndromes such as hemochromatosis, sarcoidosis, or amyloidosis. The relatively normal liver histology and normal hepatic hemodynamics do not suggest a significant primary intrinsic liver disease. The two uncles with cirrhosis could suggest a heritable liver disease, although cirrhosis in multiple family members is frequently accounted for by shared habits such as alcohol consumption or excessive caloric intake. Liver disorders with a genetic component, such as hemochromatosis, Wilson's disease, and alpha-1-antitrypsin deficiency are mostly autosomal recessive, which would make this pattern of transmission unusual. Furthermore, aside from hemochromatosis, these genetic hepatic disorders have few cardiac manifestations. Right-sided congestion and amiodarone appear to be the most likely explanations of his liver abnormalities.

Pulmonary function testing revealed normal lung volumes without obstruction, but the diffusing capacity for carbon monoxide was substantially reduced. Computed tomography of the chest identified scattered ground-glass opacities as well as small nodules with an upper lobe distribution (Fig. 16.4). Although not reported on the initial interpretation, review of a chest X-ray taken 6 months previously also demonstrated small nodules in the upper lobe distribution. Bronchoscopic examination was normal. Bronchioalveolar lavage fluid stains and cultures for bacteria, mycobacteria, *Pneumocystis*, and fungus were negative. Transbronchial biopsies of the right middle lobe had no evidence of infection, malignancy, or granulomatous inflammation. The patient continued to have progressive New York Heart Association Class IV heart failure symptoms. Repeat right heart catheterization was notable for a cardiac index of1.4 L/minute/m^2. The mean pulmonary artery pressure was 20 mm Hg. An intra-aortic balloon pump was placed for refractory cardiogenic shock.

The reduced diffusion capacity and ground-glass opacities suggest an interstitial process, which may have been missed on transbronchial biopsy because of sampling

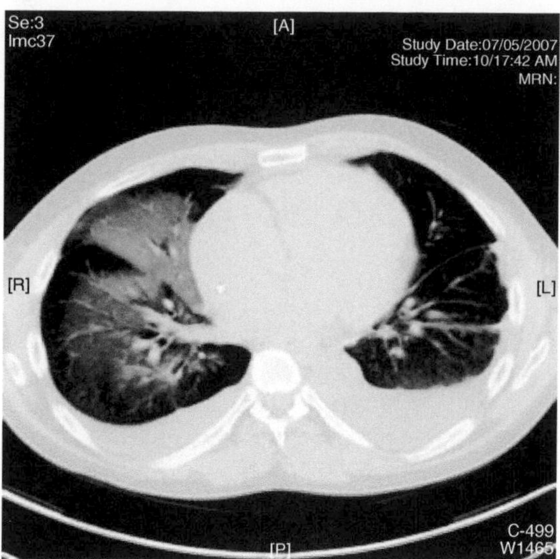

FIGURE 16.4 Computed tomography of the chest reveals asymmetrical ground-glass opacities and small nodules with an upper lobe predominance. Also shown are bilateral pleural effusions and a dilated right heart.

error. His pulmonary disease is likely another manifestation of his infiltrative cardiac disease. The constellation of cardiac, pulmonary, and hepatic involvement in the context of progressive dyspnea over 2 years is suggestive of sarcoidosis, although the absence of hilar lymphadenopathy and two biopsy specimens without granulomas argue against the diagnosis, and the effects of amiodarone on the latter two organs cannot be ignored. On the limited menu of pharmacologic treatments that may help treat this severe and progressive cardiomyopathy are steroids, which makes a diligent search for a steroid-responsive syndrome important. Therefore, despite the negative studies, sarcoidosis must be investigated to the fullest extent with either an endomyocardial biopsy or surgical lung biopsy.

The patient underwent cardiac transplantation. The native heart was found to have right ventricular thinning, which was most notable at the right ventricular outflow tract. Microscopic examination revealed extensive fibrosis and granulomatous inflammation (Fig. 16.5) with scarring typical of cardiac sarcoidosis. Six months after cardiac transplantation, the patient was doing well on prednisone, tacrolimus, and mycophenolate mofetil. Follow-up chest X-rays showed resolution of the pulmonary nodules.

COMMENTARY

Cardiomyopathy in a young person is a relatively uncommon clinical event that prompts consideration of a broad differential diagnosis that is notably different from the most common etiologies of cardiomyopathy in older adults. This case highlights the challenges of arriving at a diagnosis in the absence of a gold standard, and the greater challenges of modifying initial diagnostic impressions as new clinical data become available.

After encountering ventricular tachycardia and right ventricular dysfunction in a young patient, the clinicians arrived at the diagnosis of ARVD. This rare and progressive

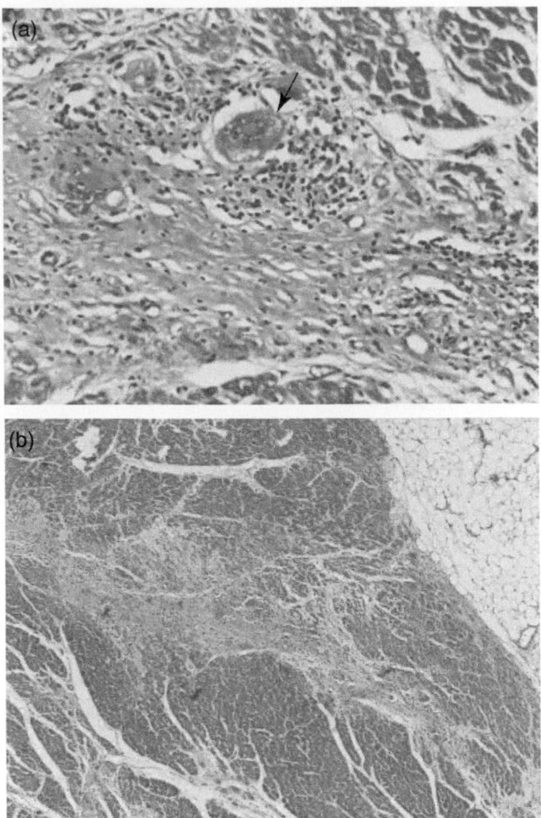

FIGURE 16.5 Microscopic examination of the patient's explanted heart demonstrated areas of chronic inflammation with (a) giant cells and (b) granulomas and extensive fibrosis.

disorder is associated with up to 20% of ventricular arrhythmias and sudden death in the young,[1,2] but can be challenging to diagnose. Despite common referrals for cardiac MRI to "exclude ARVD," cardiac MRI is not the gold standard for diagnosis and is the most common method of misdiagnosis of ARVD.[3] A diagnosis of ARVD requires the presence of 2 major, 1 major and 2 minor, or 4 minor International Task Force criteria (Table 16.1).[4,5] While the diagnostic criteria provide standardization across populations (e.g., in clinical studies), additional considerations are needed in the management of individual patients. Scoring systems serve as a tool, but the final diagnosis requires balancing such criteria with competing hypotheses. This dilemma is familiar to clinicians considering other less common conditions such as amyotrophic lateral sclerosis (World Neurology Foundation), rheumatic fever (the Jones criteria), or systemic lupus erythematosus (American College of Rheumatology). This patient's cardiac MRI findings, precordial T-wave inversions, frequent ventricular ectopy, and late potentials on a signal-averaged electrocardiogram fulfilled the International Task Force criteria for a diagnosis of ARVD. Discordant information included the right bundle branch pattern of the ventricular tachycardia, which suggested left ventricular origin, as opposed to the more common left bundle branch pattern observed in ARVD, and the absence of a family history. In addition, in the US population, only 25% of cases present with heart failure and fewer than 5% develop biventricular failure.[6] Nonetheless, this patient's imaging evidence of right ventricular structural abnormalities and dysfunction and electrocardiographic

TABLE 16.1 International Task Force Criteria for the Diagnosis of Arrhythmogenic Right Ventricular Dysplasia

	Major	Minor
I. Global and/or regional dysfunction and structural alterations	Severe dilation and reduction of right ventricular ejection fraction, localized right ventricular aneurysms	Mild right ventricular dilatation and/or reduced ejection fraction
II. Endomyocardial biopsy	Fibrofatty replacement of myocardium	—
III. Repolarization abnormalities	—	T-wave inversion in leads V1–V3 or beyond
IV. Depolarization/conduction abnormalities	Epsilon waves or localized QRS prolongation (>110 ms) in leads V1–V3	Late potentials on signal-averaged electrocardiogram
V. Arrhythmias	—	Left bundle branch block-type ventricular tachycardia (sustained and nonsustained) or frequent ventricular extra systoles (>1000/24 hours)
VI. Family history	Familial disease confirmed at necropsy or surgery	Familial history of premature sudden death (<35 years old) or clinical diagnosis based on present criteria

NOTE: A diagnosis of ARVD requires the presence of 2 major, 1 major and 2 minor, or 4 minor International Task Force criteria.

abnormalities coupled with the absence of obvious systemic disease made ARVD the logical working diagnosis.

When more widespread manifestations developed, namely, hepatic and pulmonary abnormalities, each was investigated with imaging and biopsy. Once a multisystem illness became apparent, the discussant reframed the patient's illness to include other diagnostic possibilities. In practice, it is difficult to reverse a working diagnosis despite contradictory evidence because of the common pitfall of anchoring bias. Tversky and Kahneman[7] were the first to describe the cognitive processes behind probability assessment and decision making in time-sensitive situations. Under these conditions, decision makers tend to focus on the first symptom, striking feature, or diagnosis and "anchor" subsequent probabilities to that initial presentation. Once a decision or diagnosis has been reached, clinicians tend to interpret subsequent findings in the context of the original diagnosis rather than reevaluating their initial impression. In the setting of a "known" diagnosis of ARVD, three separate diagnoses (ARVD, amiodarone-associated lung injury, and amiodarone-induced hepatic dysfunction) were considered by the treating physicians. The initial diagnosis of ARVD followed by the sequential, rather than simultaneous, manifestations of sarcoidosis made arriving at the revised diagnosis even more challenging.

Cardiac sarcoidosis can mimic ARVD and should be considered when evaluating a patient for right ventricular dysplasia.[8,9] The differential diagnosis of ARVD includes idiopathic ventricular tachycardia, myocarditis, idiopathic cardiomyopathy, and sarcoidosis. Cardiac sarcoidosis can present as ventricular ectopy, sustained ventricular arrhythmias, asymptomatic ventricular dysfunction, heart failure, or sudden death.[10] Although 25% of patients with sarcoidosis have evidence of cardiac involvement at

TABLE 16.2 Prevalence of Clinical Manifestations of Cardiac Sarcoidosis

Clinical Manifestation	Prevalence (%)
Atrioventricular block	40
Bundle branch block	40
Supraventricular tachycardia	20
Ventricular arrhythmias	25
Heart failure	25
Sudden cardiac death	35

autopsy, only 5% have clinical manifestations.[11] Those patients with clinical evidence of cardiac sarcoidosis have a wide range of clinical findings (Table 16.2). While the patient's cardiomyopathy was advanced, it is possible that earlier administration of corticosteroid therapy may have arrested his progressive biventricular failure. As clinicians, we should always remember to force ourselves to broaden our differential diagnosis when new findings become available, especially those that point to a systemic—rather than an organ-specific—disorder. In this case, while the original diagnostic findings were accurate and strongly suggested ARVD, a change of heart was needed to arrive at the ultimate diagnosis.

Key Points

1. Cardiomyopathy in a young person requires consideration of a broad differential diagnosis that is distinct from the most common etiologies of cardiomyopathy in the elderly.
2. Anchoring bias is a common pitfall in clinical decision making. When new or contradictory findings are uncovered, clinicians should reevaluate their initial impression to ensure it remains the most likely diagnosis.
3. The differential diagnosis of ARVD includes idiopathic ventricular tachycardia, right ventricular outflow tract tachycardia, myocarditis, idiopathic dilated cardiomyopathy, and sarcoidosis.

REFERENCES

1. Marcus FI, Fontaine GH, Guiraudon G, et al. Right ventricular dysplasia: A report of 24 adult cases. *Circulation*. 1982;65:384–398.
2. Thiene G, Nava A, Corrado D, Rossi L, Pennelli N. Right ventricular cardiomyopathy and sudden death in young people. *N Engl J Med*. 1988;318:129–133.
3. Bomma C, Rutberg J, Tandri H, et al. Misdiagnosis of arrhythmogenic right ventricular dysplasia/cardiomyopathy. *J Cardiovasc Electrophysiol*. 2004;15:300–306.
4. McKenna WJ, Thiene G, Nava A, et al. Diagnosis of arrhythmogenic right ventricular dysplasia/cardiomyopathy. Task Force of the Working Group Myocardial and Pericardial Disease of the European Society of Cardiology and the Scientific Council on Cardiomyopathies of the International Society and Federation of Cardiology. *Br Heart J*. 1994;71:215–218.
5. Piccini JP, Dalal D, Roguin A, et al. Predictors of appropriate implantable defibrillator therapies in patients with arrhythmogenic right ventricular dysplasia. *Heart Rhythm*. 2005;2:1188–1194.
6. Dalal D, Nasir K, Bomma C, et al. Arrhythmogenic right ventricular dysplasia: A United States experience. *Circulation*. 2005;112:3823–3832.
7. Tversky A, Kahneman D. Judgment under uncertainty: Heuristics and biases. *Science*. 1974;185: 1124–1131.

8. Tandri H, Bomma C, Calkins H. Unusual presentation of cardiac sarcoidosis. *Congest Heart Fail*. 2007;13:116–118.
9. Shiraishi J, Tatsumi T, Shimoo K, et al. Cardiac sarcoidosis mimicking right ventricular dysplasia. *Circ J*. 2003;67:169–171.
10. Koplan BA, Soejima K, Baughman K, Epstein LM, Stevenson WG. Refractory ventricular tachycardia secondary to cardiac sarcoid: Electrophysiologic characteristics, mapping, and ablation. *Heart Rhythm*. 2006;3:924–929.
11. Bargout R, Kelly RF. Sarcoid heart disease: Clinical course and treatment. *Int J Cardiol*. 2004;97:173–182.

CHAPTER **17**

MISSING THE FOREST FOR THE TREES

SATISH GOPAL
Department of Internal Medicine, Norwalk Hospital, Norwalk, Connecticut

JAMES C. PILE
Departments of Hospital Medicine and Infectious Diseases, Cleveland Clinic, Cleveland, Ohio

DANIEL J. BROTMAN
Department of Medicine, Johns Hopkins Hospital, Baltimore, Maryland

A 56-year-old woman from Colombia presented to the emergency department after 24 hours of abdominal pain. One week before, she had experienced similar pain that lasted for 4 hours and spontaneously resolved. She was nauseated but had no vomiting. She reported an unintentional 14-pound weight loss over the preceding 3 weeks. She denied fever, chills, night sweats, diarrhea, constipation, dysuria, or jaundice.

In a middle-aged woman with abdominal pain and nausea, diagnostic considerations include gallbladder disease, diseases of the bowel (such as a partial small-bowel obstruction or inflammatory conditions), hepatic or pancreatic conditions, and nongastrointestinal ailments such as cardiac ischemia. Knowing the specific location of pain, its quality, precipitating factors, and accompanying systemic symptoms may help to narrow the diagnosis. The unintentional weight loss preceding the onset of pain may be an important clue because it suggests a systemic condition, and in a South American immigrant—particularly if she has traveled recently—it is important to consider parasitic illnesses. The absence of fever makes some infections such as tuberculosis and malaria less likely. At this point, in addition to a thorough history and physical, laboratory tests should include a complete blood count (with quantification of eosinophils) and a metabolic panel with liver enzymes and albumin.

The patient described pain in the midline, just inferior to the umbilicus. The pain was constant, developed without any particular provocation, and not related to meals or exertion. There were no constitutional symptoms aside from weight loss. She had a history of bipolar disorder, hypothyroidism, osteoarthritis, and chronic sinusitis and had previously undergone cholecystectomy and abdominal hysterectomy. She was taking levothyroxine, montelukast, bupropion, oxcarbazepine, fexofenadine, meloxicam, zolpidem, and, as needed, acetaminophen. She had recently completed a 10-day course of levofloxacin for acute sinusitis. She had immigrated

Clinical Care Conundrums: Challenging Diagnoses in Hospital Medicine, First Edition.
Edited by James C. Pile, Thomas E. Baudendistel, and Brian J. Harte.

to the United States 10 years earlier and lived with her husband and daughter. She denied the use of tobacco, alcohol, or illicit drugs. She had visited Colombia 6 months earlier but had no other recent travel history.

The history of cholecystectomy makes a biliary tract process unlikely. Its location reduces the likelihood of a hepatic or pancreatic process, but I would like to see the liver enzymes, especially given her recent acetaminophen use. The comorbid illnesses—particularly her bipolar disorder—may be relevant because psychiatric illness might be associated with medication overuse or undisclosed toxic ingestions. For example, excess thyroxine might lead to weight loss while overuse of nonsteroidal anti-inflammatory drugs (NSAIDs), such as meloxicam, can cause intestinal ulceration, not only in the upper tract but also in the colon. Undisclosed ingestions may also be associated with abdominal symptoms. Her surgical history makes adhesions with a secondary partial bowel obstruction possible. With no travel outside the country in the last 6 months, exotic infections are less likely. Finally, the recent course of levofloxacin may be relevant because many antibiotics are associated with nonspecific abdominal symptoms, and *Clostridium difficile* colitis occasionally presents without diarrhea.

The patient reported taking her medications as prescribed and denied ingesting other medications. On physical examination, she had a temperature of 98.9°F, a pulse of 81 beats per minute, a blood pressure of 110/80 mm Hg, and a respiratory rate of 16 respirations per minute. She had a normal oxygen saturation while breathing ambient air. Her weight was 58 kg. There was no scleral icterus or jugular venous distension. She had a small painless ulcer involving the hard palate. Her lungs were clear to auscultation, and cardiac examination was normal. The abdomen was soft, bowel sounds were present, and there was moderate tenderness to palpation inferior to the umbilicus. There was no rebound or guarding, hepatosplenomegaly, or other masses. There was no peripheral edema and no lymphadenopathy. Neurological examination was normal.

The oral ulcer may or may not be related to the clinical presentation. Whether painful or painless, oral ulcers are ubiquitous and may be isolated or associated with a wide range of infectious and noninfectious systemic diseases. Although some systemic causes of mucocutaneous ulcers are associated with weight loss (including Crohn's disease, Behcet's disease, celiac sprue, human immunodeficiency virus [HIV], herpesviruses, syphilis, and systemic lupus erythematosus [SLE]), the lack of specificity of this finding limits its diagnostic utility. However, it is reasonable to ask whether the patient has noted frequent ulceration in the mouth or genitalia, as recurrent or severe ulcerations may narrow the diagnostic considerations. On the other hand, the focal nature of the pain inferior to the umbilicus suggests a discrete process in the abdomen or pelvis, such as an abscess, mass, or localized area of bowel inflammation. A plain abdominal film is likely to be low yield in this situation, so pursuing with computed tomography is appropriate. Not all patients with focal abdominal pain require abdominal imaging, but in the context of weight loss and persistent symptoms for more than a week, imaging is prudent in this case.

The patient denied genital ulceration but did report painless oral ulcers over the preceding months. Laboratory evaluation revealed a white-cell count of 1000/mm^3, of which 6% were neutrophils, 5% were band forms, 36% were lymphocytes, and 47% were monocytes. The absolute neutrophil count was 110/mm^3. Hemoglobin level was 10.2 g/dL with a mean corpuscular volume of 90 nm^3, and the platelet count was 151,000/mm^3. Other results of laboratory studies were sodium, 140 mmol/L; potassium, 3.8 mmol/L; chloride, 96 mmol/L; bicarbonate, 23 mmol/L; blood urea nitrogen, 13 mg/dL; creatinine, 0.4 mg/dL;

lipase, 32 U/L (normal range, 13–60); amylase, 73 U/L (normal range, 30–110); albumin, 4.0 g/dL; aspartate aminotransferase (AST), 779 U/L (normal range, 13–35); alanine aminotransferase, 330 U/L (normal range, 7–35); alkaline phosphatase, 510 U/L (normal range, 35–104); and total bilirubin, 0.9 mg/dL (normal range, 0.1–1.2). The lactate dehydrogenase level was 200 U/L (normal range, 135–214). The corrected reticulocyte count was 1.6% (normal range, 0.3–2.3), and haptoglobin was 190 mg/dL (normal range, 43–212). A direct Coombs' test was positive. The erythrocyte sedimentation rate was 113 mm/hour (normal range, 1–25). Urinalysis was normal without evidence of protein or blood.

Laboratory abnormalities include elevated transaminases and alkaline phosphatase, a markedly elevated erythrocyte sedimentation rate, and profound leukopenia with neutropenia. The patient is anemic, which may elevate the sedimentation rate but not typically to this degree. The patient is not febrile, but if she were to develop fever, treatment using empiric antibiotics would be prudent. The normal albumin and bilirubin suggest that hepatic synthetic and excretory functions remain intact. Although the direct Coombs test is positive, the reticulocyte and lactate dehydrogenase levels argue against brisk hemolysis; this abnormality may simply be a marker of nonspecific immune activation. A variety of infections can cause neutropenia and liver enzyme abnormalities, including parasites (malaria or leishmaniasis), viruses (cytomegalovirus or Epstein–Barr virus [EBV]), tick-borne bacterial infections (ehrlichiosis or rickettsial infection), and granulomatous infections (tuberculosis). Malignant infiltration of the reticuloendothelial system can also lead to cytopenias and liver enzyme abnormalities. Autoimmunity remains a consideration, as SLE may lead to cytopenias, oral ulcers, and nonspecific immune phenomena. Rather than ordering a large number of blood tests, I favor a targeted approach with abdominal computed tomography followed by biopsy of either the liver or bone marrow.

Chest radiography revealed no abnormalities. Computed tomography of the chest, abdomen, and pelvis with intravenous and oral contrast demonstrated concentric wall thickening of the transverse colon, but no evidence of obstruction or free air. The patient was treated with intravenous fluids, morphine, and cefepime. Bone marrow biopsy was performed, which demonstrated a hypercellular marrow with increased myeloid precursors and a left shift and megakaryocytic hyperplasia. Flow cytometry revealed no abnormally restricted clonal populations. A concerted search for an infectious etiology of the patient's neutropenia was unrevealing, including tests for HIV, cytomegalovirus, hepatitis A, hepatitis B, hepatitis C, *Mycoplasma pneumoniae*, EBV, and parvovirus B19.

I hope blood cultures were drawn prior to the initiation of antibiotics. Hypercellularity of the bone marrow in the context of leukopenia raises concern that white blood cells are being destroyed peripherally. Autoimmunity against neutrophils can be transiently induced by viruses such as HIV, hepatitis B, and EBV, but these infections have been excluded. Testing for antinuclear antibodies (ANAs) is reasonable. A normal-sized spleen on the abdominal CT excludes hypersplenism. Colonic thickening can be associated with infection, ischemia, inflammatory bowel disease, and malignancy. The question is whether the colonic thickening is part of the same disease process causing the leukopenia and liver enzyme elevation or whether it represents a secondary infectious process in the setting of neutropenia (such as *C. difficile* infection or typhlitis). Testing for stool pathogens (including ova and parasites) is certainly appropriate, and consideration of a colonoscopy with biopsy is reasonable, provided that appropriate antimicrobial coverage remains in place.

Blood cultures obtained prior to starting antibiotics were negative. The patient's abdominal pain improved, and she was discharged home to have close follow-up with a hematologist. The results of her liver function tests improved, and her absolute neutrophil count was 230/mm^3 at the time of discharge. Her neutropenia was believed to be secondary to peripheral destruction from a viral, drug-mediated, or autoimmune process. Oxcarbazepine (Trileptal) was discontinued, as it was believed to be the medication most likely to be responsible. She returned to the hospital 3 days later with recurrence of her abdominal pain and diarrhea. She remained afebrile. Additional history revealed arthralgias over the previous 2 months, mild alopecia, and prior symptoms suggestive of Raynaud's phenomenon. Stool studies failed to establish an infectious etiology for the diarrhea, and her continued neutropenia responded appropriately to treatment with subcutaneous filgrastim. Colonoscopy could be performed only to the hepatic flexure and revealed no abnormalities. A serologic test for ANAs was positive at a titer of 1:640 in a homogenous pattern, and a test for antineutrophil cytoplasmic antibodies was negative. Complement levels were normal, and tests for cryoglobulins, rapid plasma reagin, anticardiolipin antibody, lupus anticoagulant, rheumatoid factor, and antibodies to extractable nuclear antigens were all negative.

Raynaud's phenomenon is consistent with lupus. Double-stranded DNA antibodies should be sent, although the urine did not demonstrate protein or an active sediment. Systemic sclerosis and the CREST syndrome are strongly associated with Raynaud's phenomenon and high-titer ANA, but the patient does not have sclerodactyly, which is generally the earliest skin involvement. Autoimmune hepatitis is often associated with high-titer ANA but does not fit this clinical picture. Given that the patient's presentation included segmental bowel wall thickening and a transient but marked liver enzyme elevation with AST predominance, I am concerned about vasculitis of the abdominal vasculature and would strongly consider a mesenteric angiogram.

To exclude mesenteric vasculitis, the patient underwent magnetic resonance angiography of the abdomen, the results of which were normal. A repeat test for ANAs was positive at a titer of 1:2560 in a uniform pattern. A test for anti-double-stranded DNA was positive at 1370 U/mL. The patient was diagnosed with SLE and probable lupus enteritis, and therapy with oral prednisone (10 mg daily) and hydroxychloroquine was initiated. She had prompt improvement in her abdominal pain and was discharged home. Five months later she developed proteinuria and underwent a renal biopsy, which showed minor, nonspecific glomerular abnormalities, suggesting possible mild lupus nephritis. Eight months after her initial presentation, she remains free of abdominal pain and has regained the weight she had initially lost. Her oral ulcers have resolved, and her blood counts have normalized. Her serum creatinine has remained normal. She is now maintained on prednisone (15 mg daily), hydroxychloroquine, and mycophenolate mofetil.

COMMENTARY

A diagnosis of SLE provided a unifying explanation for the patient's findings. Indeed, she manifested 4 of the 11 American College of Rheumatology criteria for SLE (oral ulcers, leukopenia, positive anti-DNA, and positive ANA), meeting criteria for a definite diagnosis of SLE. She additionally had multiple other features suggestive of lupus including Raynaud's phenomenon, arthralgias, alopecia, mild thrombocytopenia, and a positive

Coombs' test (although the normal reticulocyte count, lactate dehydrogenase, and haptoglobin were most consistent with anemia of a chronic disease).

The protean manifestations of SLE can present significant diagnostic challenges. In this case, physicians were immediately drawn to the patient's acute abdominal pain and severe neutropenia and failed to recognize more subtle disease manifestations that may have aided in establishing a unifying diagnosis sooner. The initial history and review of systems did not disclose arthralgias, alopecia, or Raynaud's phenomenon. In an era of increasing use of hospitalists, which creates potential discontinuity between inpatient and outpatient physicians, a thorough history and review of systems may be particularly important in diagnosing acute manifestations of chronic systemic disease. Inpatient physicians may be overly focused on the small subset of acute complaints leading to hospitalization, without considering the larger constellation of symptoms that may facilitate accurate diagnosis. Our discussant quickly recognized the multisystem nature of the patient's illness and appropriately focused on infectious, neoplastic, and autoimmune categories of disease as being most likely. When infectious and neoplastic conditions were excluded with reasonable certainty, a directed serologic investigation for autoimmune disease was requested, culminating in a diagnosis of SLE.

Involvement of the skin as well as hematologic, renal, and musculoskeletal systems in SLE is commonly recognized, whereas gastrointestinal involvement is perceived to occur much less frequently. However, abdominal pain occurs in up to 40% of patients with lupus.[1–4] Abdominal pain in lupus patients can arise from non-lupus-related conditions as well as lupus-related entities, including serositis, mesenteric vasculitis with or without infarction, mesenteric thrombosis, pancreatitis, inflammatory bowel disease, and adverse medication effects including peptic ulcer disease. Abnormal liver chemistries, as seen in our patient, occur in 20%–50% of patients with lupus and may be due to lupus hepatitis, concomitant autoimmune hepatitis, or medications including NSAIDs.[5,6] Oral ulcers and leukopenia are likewise common in SLE, with each seen in up to half of patients.[4,7,8] Leukopenia in SLE may be a result of neutropenia, lymphocytopenia, or both. However, severe neutropenia (ie, absolute count less than 500/μL), as seen in this patient, is more often a result of myelotoxicity from immunosuppressive therapy, rather than SLE itself.[9]

Lupus enteritis represents bowel microischemia from small-vessel arteritis or venulitis that often is not evident on conventional mesenteric angiography.[4,10,11] The reported prevalence of intestinal vasculitis in patients with SLE varies widely, depending on the characteristics of lupus patients sampled in individual studies. Intestinal vasculitis affects 0.2%–0.5% of SLE patients in general,[4,12] whereas among SLE patients with active disease and an acute abdomen, vasculitis has been reported in up to 53% of patients.[10] Antiphospholipid antibodies, antibodies to extractable nuclear antigens, the SLE Disease Activity Index, complement levels, erythrocyte sedimentation rate, C-reactive protein, and anti-double-stranded DNA do not reliably differentiate lupus enteritis from acute abdominal pain due to other etiologies in patients with SLE.[11] However, a concomitant drop in the white blood cell count at the onset of symptoms may be useful in distinguishing lupus enteritis from other causes of acute abdominal pain among lupus patients.[11] Computed tomography findings consistent with lupus enteritis are nonspecific and include bowel wall thickening, submucosal edema (e.g., target sign), dilatation of intestinal segments, engorgement of mesenteric vessels, and increased attenuation of mesenteric fat.[13] Colonoscopy may reveal areas of ischemia and ulceration, and biopsy can confirm intestinal vasculitis. However, intestinal involvement may be segmental, and pathologic confirmation may be difficult. Contrast enema, gallium scanning, and indium-labeled white-cell scanning may be useful, but lack specificity. No controlled trials to date have evaluated the optimal therapy for lupus enteritis, but pulsed methylprednisolone is often recommended.[4] Cyclophosphamide, azathioprine, methotrexate, and cyclosporine have also been used as adjunctive agents. Patients may progress to intestinal infarction and perforation, which augurs a poor prognosis, and early surgical exploration should be considered in severely ill patients.[10] Death may occur in more than two-thirds of patients whose disease progresses to intestinal perforation.[1]

In summary, a multisystem disease such as SLE requires a comprehensive history, physical exam, and review of systems to establish a correct diagnosis. In our case, an extensive evaluation was necessary to exclude other etiologies of abdominal pain and systemic illness, particularly as infectious and neoplastic conditions occur far more often than lupus enteritis in the general population. However, profound laboratory abnormalities may have preoccupied the attention of treating physicians, leading them to overlook less obvious but important historical and physical findings suggestive of SLE. The cohesively abnormal "forest" may thus have been obscured by erratically abnormal individual "trees."

Key Points

1. Abdominal pain occurs in up to 40% of patients with SLE, but mesenteric vasculitis is the cause in fewer than 1%.
2. Enteric vasculitis due to SLE is challenging to diagnose. Serologic tests and routine imaging results are nonspecific, and angiography may be normal. Diagnosis relies on searching for other clues to systemic involvement by SLE and reasonably excluding alternative disorders.

REFERENCES

1. Hoffman, BI, Katz, WA. The gastrointestinal manifestations of systemic lupus erythematosus: A review of the literature. *Semin Arthritis Rheum*. 1980;9:237.
2. Zizic TM, Classen JN, Stevens MB. Acute abdominal complications of systemic lupus erythematosus and polyarteritis nodosa. *Am J Med*. 1982;73:525–531.
3. Jovaisas A, Kraag G. Acute gastrointestinal manifestations of systemic lupus erythematosus. *Can J Surg*. 1987;30:185–188.
4. Sultan SM, Ioannou Y, Isenberg DA. A review of gastrointestinal manifestations of systemic lupus erythematosus. *Rheumatology*. 1999;38:917–932.
5. Youssef WI, Tavill AS. Connective tissue disease and the liver. *J Clin Gastroenterol*. 2002;35:345–349.
6. Runyon BA, LaBrecque DR, Anuras S. The spectrum of liver disease in systemic lupus erythematosus: Report of 33 histologically-proved cases and review of the literature. *Am J Med*. 1980;69:187–194.
7. Budman DR, Steinberg AD. Hematologic aspects of systemic lupus erythematosus: Current concepts. *Ann Intern Med*. 1977;86:220–229.
8. Nossent JC, Swaak AJ. Prevalence and significance of hematological abnormalities in patients with systemic lupus erythematosus. *Q J Med*. 1991;80:605–12.
9. Martinez-Banos D, Crispin JC, Lazo-Langner A, et al. Moderate and severe neutropenia in patients with systemic lupus erythematosus. *Rheumatology*. 2006;45:994–998.
10. Medina F, Ayala A, Lara LJ, et al. Acute abdomen in systemic lupus erythematosus: The importance of early laparotomy. *Am J Med*. 1997;103:100–105.
11. Lee C, Ahn MS, Lee EY, et al. Acute abdominal pain in systemic lupus erythematosus: Focus on lupus enteritis (gastrointestinal vasculitis). *Ann Rheum Dis*. 2002;61:547–550.
12. Drenkard C, Villa AR, Reyes E, et al. Vasculitis in systemic lupus erythematosus. *Lupus*. 1997;6:235–242.
13. Byun JY, Ha HK, Yu SY, et al. CT features of systemic lupus erythematosus in patients with acute abdominal pain: Emphasis on ischemic bowel disease. *Radiology*. 1999;211:203–209.

CHAPTER **18**

A PAIN IN THE BONE

JOHN FANI SROUR
Division of General Medicine and Primary Care, Beth Israel Deaconess Medical Center, Harvard Medical School, Boston, Massachusetts

JULIA BRAZA
Division of Pathology, Beth Israel Deaconess Medical Center, Harvard Medical School, Boston, Massachusetts

GERALD W. SMETANA
Division of General Medicine and Primary Care, Beth Israel Deaconess Medical Center, Harvard Medical School, Boston, Massachusetts

A 71-year-old man presented to a hospital with a 1-week history of fatigue, polyuria, and polydipsia. He also reported pain in his back, hips, and ribs, in addition to frequent falls, intermittent confusion, constipation, and a weight loss of 10 pounds over the last 2 weeks. He denied cough, shortness of breath, chest pain, fever, night sweats, headache, and focal weakness.

Polyuria, which is often associated with polydipsia, can be arbitrarily defined as a urine output exceeding 3 L per day. After excluding osmotic diuresis due to uncontrolled diabetes mellitus, the three major causes of polyuria are primary polydipsia, central diabetes insipidus, and nephrogenic diabetes insipidus. Approximately 30%–50% of cases of central diabetes insipidus are idiopathic; however, primary or secondary brain tumors or infiltrative diseases involving the hypothalamic-pituitary region need to be considered in this 71-year-old man. The most common causes of nephrogenic diabetes insipidus in adults are chronic lithium ingestion, hypokalemia, and hypercalcemia. The patient describes symptoms that can result from severe hypercalcemia, including fatigue, confusion, constipation, polyuria, and polydipsia.

The patient's past medical history included long-standing, insulin-requiring type 2 diabetes with associated complications including coronary artery disease, transient ischemic attacks, proliferative retinopathy, peripheral diabetic neuropathy, and nephropathy. Seven years prior to presentation, he received a cadaveric renal transplant that was complicated by the BK virus (polyomavirus) nephropathy and secondary hyperparathyroidism. Three years after his transplant surgery, he developed squamous cell carcinoma of the skin, which was treated with local surgical resection. Two years after that, he developed stage I laryngeal cancer of the glottis and received laser surgery, and since then, he had been considered disease-free. He also had a history of hypertension, hypercholesterolemia, osteoporosis, and depression. His medications included aspirin, amlodipine, metoprolol

Clinical Care Conundrums: Challenging Diagnoses in Hospital Medicine, First Edition.
Edited by James C. Pile, Thomas E. Baudendistel, and Brian J. Harte.

succinate, valsartan, furosemide, simvastatin, insulin, prednisone, sirolimus, and sulfamethoxazole/trimethoprim. He was a married psychiatrist. He denied tobacco use and reported occasional alcohol use.

The prolonged immunosuppressive therapy that is required following organ transplantation carries a markedly increased risk of subsequent development of malignant tumors, including cancers of the lips and skin, lymphoproliferative disorders, and bronchogenic carcinoma. Primary brain lymphoma resulting in central diabetes insipidus would be unlikely in the absence of headache or focal weakness. An increased risk of lung cancer occurs in recipients of heart and lung transplants, and to a much lesser degree, in recipients of kidney transplants. However, metastatic lung cancer is less likely in the absence of respiratory symptoms and smoking history (present in approximately 90% of all lung cancers). Nephrogenic diabetes insipidus, in its mild form, is relatively common in elderly patients with acute or chronic renal insufficiency because of a reduction in maximum urinary concentrating ability. On the other hand, this alone does not explain his remaining symptoms. The "instinctive" diagnosis in this case is tertiary hyperparathyroidism due to progression of untreated secondary hyperparathyroidism. This causes hypercalcemia, nephrogenic diabetes insipidus, and significant bone pain related to renal osteodystrophy.

On physical exam, the patient appeared chronically ill, but was in no acute distress. He weighed 197.6 pounds, and his height was 70.5 inches. He was afebrile with a blood pressure of 146/82 mm Hg, a heart rate of 76 beats per minute, a respiratory rate of 12 breaths per minute, and an oxygen saturation of 97% while breathing room air. He had no generalized lymphadenopathy. Thyroid examination was unremarkable. Examination of the lungs, heart, abdomen, and lower extremities was normal. The rectal examination revealed no masses or prostate nodules; a test for fecal occult blood was negative. He had loss of sensation to light touch and vibration in the feet with absent Achilles deep tendon reflexes. He had a poorly healing surgical wound on his forehead at the site of his prior skin cancer, but no rash or other lesions. There was no joint swelling or erythema. There were tender points over the cervical, thoracic, and lumbar spine; on multiple ribs; and on the pelvic rims.

Perhaps of greatest importance is the lack of lymphadenopathy, organomegaly, or other findings suggestive of diffuse lymphoproliferative disease. His multifocal bone tenderness is concerning for renal osteodystrophy, multiple myeloma, or primary or metastatic bone disease. Cancers in men that metastasize to the bone usually originate from the prostate, lung, kidney, or thyroid gland. In any case, his physical examination did not reveal an enlarged, asymmetric, or a nodular prostate or thyroid gland. I recommend a chest film to rule out primary lung malignancy and a basic laboratory evaluation.

A complete blood count showed a normocytic anemia with a hemoglobin of 8.7 g/dL and a hematocrit of 25%. Other laboratory tests revealed the following values: sodium, 139 mmol/L; potassium, 4.1 mmol/L; blood urea nitrogen, 70 mg/dL; creatinine, 3.5 mg/dL (most recent value 2 months ago was 1.9 mg/dL); total calcium, 13.2 mg/dL (normal range, 8.5–10.5 mg/dL); phosphate, 5.3 mg/dL; magnesium, 2.5 mg/dL; total bilirubin, 0.5 mg/dL; alkaline phosphatase, 130 U/L; aspartate aminotransferase, 28 U/L; alanine aminotransferase, 19 U/L; albumin, 3.5 g/dL; and lactate dehydrogenase (LDH), 1258 IU/L (normal range, 105–333 IU/L). A chest radiograph was normal.

The most important laboratory findings are severe hypercalcemia, acute-on-chronic renal failure, and anemia. Hypercalcemia most commonly results from malignancy or hyperparathyroidism. Less frequently, hypercalcemia may result from sarcoidosis, vitamin D intoxication, or hyperthyroidism. The degree of hypercalcemia is useful diagnostically, as hyperparathyroidism commonly results in mild hypercalcemia (serum calcium concentration often below 11 mg/dL). Values above 13 mg/dL are unusual in hyperparathyroidism and are most often due to malignancy. Malignancy is often evident clinically by the time it causes hypercalcemia, and patients with hypercalcemia due to malignancy are more often symptomatic than those with hyperparathyroidism. Additionally, localized bone pain and weight loss do not result from hypercalcemia itself and their presence also raises concern for malignancy.

Nonmelanoma skin cancer is the most common cancer occurring after transplantation but does not cause hypercalcemia. Squamous cancers of the head and neck can rarely cause hypercalcemia due to secretion of parathyroid hormone (PTH)-related peptide; however, his early-stage laryngeal cancer and the expected high likelihood of cure argue against this possibility. Osteolytic metastases account for approximately 20% of cases of hypercalcemia of malignancy (Table 18.1). Prostate cancer rarely results in hypercalcemia since bone metastases are predominantly osteoblastic, whereas metastatic non-small-cell lung cancer, thyroid cancer, and kidney cancer more commonly cause hypercalcemia due to osteolytic bone lesions. Total alkaline phosphatase has been traditionally used to assess the osteoblastic component of bone remodeling. Its normal level tends to predict a negative bone scan and supports the likelihood of lytic lesions. Post-transplantation lymphoproliferative disorders (PTLDs), which include a wide range of syndromes, can rarely result in hypercalcemia. I am also worried about the possibility of

TABLE 18.1 Malignancies Associated with Hypercalcemia

Osteolytic Metastases
Breast cancer
Multiple myeloma
Lymphoma
Leukemia
Humoral Hypercalcemia (PTH-Related Protein)
Squamous cell carcinomas
Renal carcinomas
Bladder carcinoma
Breast cancer
Ovarian carcinoma
Leukemia
Lymphoma
1,25-Dihydroxyvitamin D Secretion
Lymphoma
Ovarian dysgerminomas
Ectopic PTH Secretion (Rare)
Ovarian carcinoma
Lung carcinomas
Neuroectodermal tumor
Thyroid papillary carcinoma
Rhabdomyosarcoma
Pancreatic cancer

Abbreviation: PTH, parathyroid hormone.

multiple myeloma, as he has the classic triad of hypercalcemia, bone pain, and subacute kidney injury.

The first purpose of laboratory evaluation is to differentiate PTH-mediated hypercalcemia (primary and tertiary hyperparathyroidism) from non-PTH-mediated hypercalcemia (primarily malignancy, hyperthyroidism, vitamin D intoxication, and granulomatous disease). The production of vitamin D metabolites, PTH-related protein, or hypercalcemia from osteolysis in these latter cases results in suppressed PTH levels.

In case of severe elevations of calcium, the initial goals of treatment are directed toward fluid resuscitation with normal saline and, unless contraindicated, the immediate institution of bisphosphonate therapy. A loop diuretic such as furosemide is often used, but a recent review concluded that there is little evidence to support its use in this setting.

The patient was admitted and treated with intravenous saline and furosemide. Additional laboratory evaluation revealed normal levels of prostate-specific antigen and thyroid-stimulating hormone. PTH was 44 pg/mL (the most recent value was 906 pg/mL, which was 8 years ago; normal range, 15–65 pg/mL) and beta-2 microglobulin (B2M) was 8 mg/L (normal range, 0.8–2.2 mg/L).

The normal PTH level makes tertiary hyperparathyroidism unlikely and points toward non-PTH-related hypercalcemia. An elevated B2M level may occur in patients with chronic graft rejection, renal tubular dysfunction, dialysis-related amyloidosis, multiple myeloma, or lymphoma. LDH is often elevated in patients with multiple myeloma and lymphoma, but this is not a specific finding. The next laboratory test would be measurement of PTH-related protein and vitamin D metabolites, as these tests can differentiate between the causes of non-PTH mediated hypercalcemia.

Serum concentrations of the vitamin D metabolites, 25-hydroxyvitamin D (calcidiol), and 1,25-dihydroxyvitamin D (calcitriol), were low-normal. PTH-related protein was not detected.

The marked elevation of serum LDH and B2M, the relatively suppressed PTH level, combined with undetectable PTH-related protein suggest multiple myeloma or lymphoma as the likely cause of the patient's clinical presentation. The combination of hypercalcemia and multifocal bone pain makes multiple myeloma the leading diagnosis, as hypercalcemia is uncommon in patients with lymphoma, especially at the time of initial clinical presentation.

I would proceed with serum and urine protein electrophoresis (SPEP and UPEP, respectively) and a skeletal survey. If these tests do not confirm the diagnosis of multiple myeloma, I would order a noncontrast computed tomography (CT) of the chest and abdomen and a magnetic resonance imaging (MRI) of the spine. In addition, I would like to monitor his response to the intravenous saline and furosemide.

Forty-eight hours after presentation, repeat serum calcium and creatinine levels were 11.3 mg/dL and 2.9 mg/dL, respectively. He received salmon calcitonin 4 U/kg every 12 hours. Pamidronate was avoided because of his kidney disease. His confusion resolved. He received intravenous morphine intermittently to alleviate his bone pain.

The SPEP revealed a monoclonal immunoglobulin G (IgG) lambda (light chain) spike representing roughly 3% (200 mg/dL) of total protein. His serum immunoglobulin levels were normal. The UPEP was negative for monoclonal immunoglobulin and Bence–Jones protein. The skeletal survey revealed marked osteopenia, and the bone scan was normal. An MRI of the spine showed multiple round lesions in the cervical, thoracic, and lumbar spine (Fig. 18.1). A CT of the

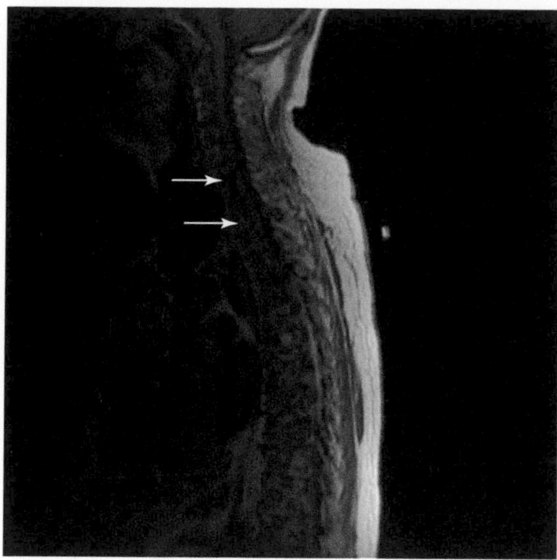

FIGURE 18.1 An MRI image of the thoracic spine showing multiple, diffuse round bone lesions (arrows).

chest showed similar bone lesions in the ribs and pelvis. A CT of the abdomen and chest neither suggested any primary malignancy nor showed thoracic or abdominal lymphadenopathy.

The lack of lymphadenopathy, splenomegaly, or a visceral mass by CT imaging and physical examination, along with the normal PSA level, exclude most common forms of non-Hodgkin lymphoma and bone metastasis from solid tumors. In multiple myeloma, cytokines secreted by plasma cells suppress osteoblast activity; therefore, while discrete lytic bone lesions are apparent on skeletal survey, the bone scan is typically normal. The absence of lytic lesions, normal serum immunoglobulin levels, and unremarkable UPEP make multiple myeloma or light-chain deposition disease a less likely diagnosis.

Typically, primary lymphoma of the bone produces increased uptake with bone scanning. However, because primary lymphoma of the bone is one of the least common primary skeletal malignancies and varies widely in appearance on imaging, confident diagnosis based on imaging alone usually is not possible.

PTLD refers to a syndrome that ranges from a self-limited form of lymphoproliferation to an aggressive disseminated disease. Although the patient is at risk for PTLD, isolated bone involvement has only rarely been reported.

Primary lymphoma of the bone and PTLD are my leading diagnoses in this patient. At this point, I recommend a bone marrow biopsy and biopsy of an easily accessible representative bone lesion with special staining for Epstein–Barr virus (EBV) (EBV-encoded RNA [EBER] and latent membrane protein 1 [LMP1]). I expect this test to provide a definitive diagnosis. As 95% of PTLD cases are induced by infection with EBV, information regarding pretransplantation EBV status of the patient and the donor, current EBV status of the patient, and type and intensity of immunosuppression at the time of transplantation would be very helpful to determine their likelihood.

Seventy-two hours after presentation, his serum calcium level normalized and most of his symptoms improved. Calcitonin was discontinued, and he was maintained on oral hydration. On hospital day 5, he underwent CT-guided bone biopsy of the L4 vertebral body, which showed large aggregates of atypical lymphoid cells

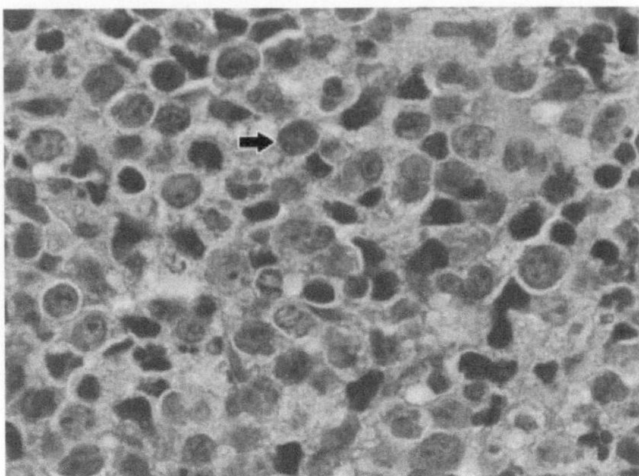

FIGURE 18.2 L4 biopsy: H&E (hematoxylin and eosin) stain (magnification ×100). The biopsy shows large aggregates of atypical lymphoid cells (arrow) that are medium in size, with vesicular chromatin, multiple prominent nucleoli, and highly lobulated nuclear membranes.

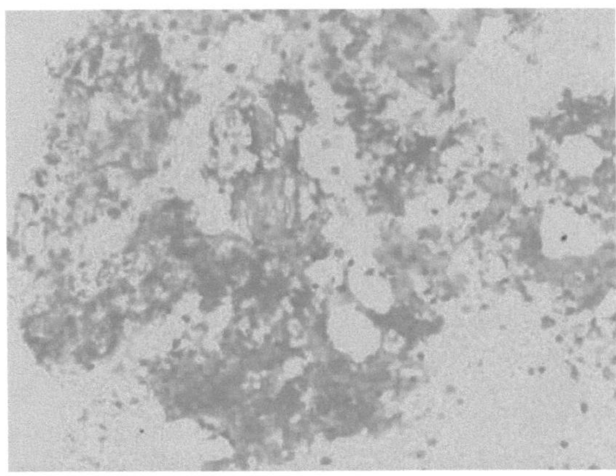

FIGURE 18.3 L4 biopsy: EBER staining (magnification ×40), demonstrating that the infiltrate is negative. **Abbreviation**: EBER, EBV-encoded RNA.

(Fig. 18.2). These cells were predominantly B cells interspersed with small reactive T cells. The cells did not express EBV LMP1 or EBER (Fig. 18.3). On hospital day 7, he underwent a bone marrow biopsy, which revealed similar large atypical lymphoid cells that comprised the majority of the marrow space (Fig. 18.4). By immunohistochemistry, these cells brightly expressed the pan B-cell marker, CD20, and coexpressed bcl-2. EBER and LMP1 were also negative. A flow cytometry of the bone marrow demonstrated a lambda light-chain restriction within the B lymphocytes.

The medical records indicated that the patient had positive pretransplantation EBV serologies. He received a regimen based on sirolimus, mycophenolate mofetil, and prednisone, and did not receive high doses of induction or maintenance immunosuppressive therapy.

The biopsy results established a diagnosis of diffuse large B-cell lymphoma of the bone. PTLD is unlikely, given his positive pretransplantation EBV status, the late onset of his disease (6 years after transplantation), the isolated bone involvement, and the negative EBER and LMP1 tests.

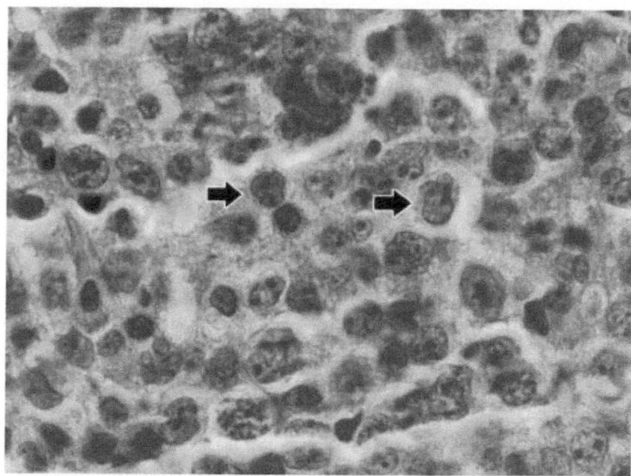

FIGURE 18.4 Bone marrow trephine core biopsy: H&E (hematoxylin and eosin) stain (magnification ×100), demonstrating similar cellular morphology to L4 lesion, with atypical cells (arrows) having convoluted nuclear membrane.

The patient was discharged and was readmitted 1 week later for induction chemotherapy with etoposide, vincristine, doxorubicin, cyclophosphamide, and prednisone [EPOCH]–Rituxan (rituximab). Over the next several months, he received 6 cycles of chemotherapy, his hypercalcemia resolved, and his back pain improved.

COMMENTARY

Hypercalcemia is among the most common causes of nephrogenic diabetes insipidus in adults.[1] A urinary concentrating defect usually becomes clinically apparent if the plasma calcium concentration is persistently above 11 mg/dL.[1] This defect is generally reversible with correction of the hypercalcemia but may persist in patients in whom interstitial nephritis has induced permanent medullary damage. The mechanism by which the concentrating defect occurs is incompletely understood but may be related to impairments in sodium chloride reabsorption in the thick ascending limb and in the ability of antidiuretic hormone to increase water permeability in the collecting tubules.[1]

Although hypercalcemia in otherwise healthy outpatients is usually due to primary hyperparathyroidism, malignancy is more often responsible for hypercalcemia in hospitalized patients.[2] While the signs and symptoms of hypercalcemia are similar regardless of the cause, several clinical features may help distinguish the etiology of hypercalcemia. For instance, the presence of tachycardia, warm skin, thinning of the hair, stare and lid lag, and widened pulse pressure points toward hypercalcemia related to hyperthyroidism. In addition, risk factors and comorbidities guide the diagnostic process. For example, low-level hypercalcemia in an asymptomatic postmenopausal woman with a normal physical examination suggests primary hyperparathyroidism. In contrast, hypercalcemia in a transplant patient raises concern of malignancy, including PTLDs.[3,4]

PTLDs are uncommon causes of hypercalcemia but are among the most serious and potentially fatal complications of chronic immunosuppression in transplant recipients.[5] They occur in 1.9% of patients after kidney transplantation. The lymphoproliferative disorders occurring after transplantation have different characteristics from those that occur in the general population. Non-Hodgkin lymphoma accounts for 65% of lymphomas in the general population, compared to 93% in transplant recipients.[5,6] The pathogenesis of PTLD appears to be related to B-cell proliferation induced by infection with EBV in the setting of chronic immunosuppression.[6] Therefore, there is an increased frequency of PTLD among transplant recipients who are EBV seronegative at the time of operation. These patients, who have no preoperative immunity to EBV, usually acquire the infection from the donor. The level of immunosuppression (intensity and type) influences PTLD rates as well. The disease typically occurs within 12 months of transplantation and in two-thirds of cases involves extranodal sites. Among these sites, the gastrointestinal tract is involved in about 26% of cases and the central nervous system in about 27%. Isolated bone involvement is exceedingly rare.[5,6]

Primary lymphoma of the bone is another rare cause of hypercalcemia and accounts for less than 5% of all primary bone tumors.[7] The majority of cases are of the non-Hodgkin's type, characterized as diffuse large B-cell lymphomas, with peak occurrence in the sixth to seventh decades of life.[8] The classic imaging findings of primary lymphoma of the bone are a solitary metadiaphyseal lesion with a layered periosteal reaction on plain radiographs, and corresponding surrounding soft tissue mass on MRI.[9] Less commonly, primary lymphoma of the bone can be multifocal with diffuse osseous involvement and variable radiographic appearances, as in this case. Most series have reported that the long bones are affected most frequently (especially the femur), although a large series showed equal numbers of cases presenting in the long bones and the spine.[7-12]

In order to diagnose primary lymphoma of the bone, it is necessary to exclude nodal or disseminated disease by physical examination and imaging. As plain films are often normal, bone scan or MRI of clinically affected areas is necessary to establish the disease extent.[9] Distinguishing primary bone lymphomas (PLBs) from other bone tumors is important because PLB has a better response to therapy and a better prognosis.[10,11]

Randomized trials addressing treatment options for PLB are not available. Historically, PLB was treated with radiotherapy alone with good local control. However, the rate of distant relapses was relatively high. Currently, chemotherapy with or without radiation therapy is preferred; 5-year survival is approximately 70% after combined therapy.[10,11]

In this case, symptomatic hypercalcemia, a history of transplantation, marked elevation of both LDH and B2M, and a normal PTH level all pointed toward malignancy. In a patient with diffuse osteopenia and hypercalcemia, clinicians must consider multiple myeloma and other lymphoproliferative disorders; the absence of osteoblastic or osteolytic lesions and a normal alkaline phosphatase do not rule out these diagnoses. When the results of SPEP and UPEP exclude multiple myeloma, the next investigation should be a bone biopsy to exclude PLB, an uncommon cause of anemia, hypercalcemia, and osteopenic, painful bones.

Key Points

1. Normal total alkaline phosphatase does not exclude primary or metastatic bone malignancy. While a normal level tends to predict a negative bone scan, further diagnostic tests are needed to exclude bone malignancy if high clinical suspicion exists.
2. The degree of hypercalcemia is useful diagnostically; values above 13 mg/dL are most often due to malignancy.
3. PTLDs occur in about 2% of patients who have undergone kidney transplant, usually within a year of the transplant, and typically in patients who were EBV seronegative prior to transplantation.
4. While rare, PLB can be considered in patients with hypercalcemia and bone pain, along with the more common diagnoses of multiple myeloma and metastatic bone disease.

REFERENCES

1. Rose BD, Post TW. *Clinical physiology of acid-base and electrolyte disorders*. 5th ed. New York: McGraw-Hill; 2001:754–758.
2. LeBoff MS, Mikulec KH. Hypercalcemia: Clinical manifestations, pathogenesis, diagnosis, and management. In: Favus MJ, ed. *Primer on the Metabolic Bone Diseases and Disorders of Mineral Metabolism*. 5th ed. Washington, DC: American Society for Bone and Mineral Research; 2003:225–230.
3. Hiesse C, Rieu P, Kriaa F, et al. Malignancy after renal transplantation: Analysis of incidence and risk factors in 1700 patients followed during a 25-year period. *Transplant Proc*. 1997;29:831–833.
4. Stewart AF, Broadus AE. Malignancy-associated hypercalcemia. In: DeGroot L, Jameson LJ, eds. *Endocrinology*. 4th ed. Philadelphia, PA: Saunders; 2001:1093–1100.
5. Preiksaitis JK, Keay S. Diagnosis and management of posttransplant lymphoproliferative disorder in solid-organ transplant recipients. *Clin Infect Dis*. 2001;33(Suppl 1):S38–S46.
6. Paya CV, Fung JJ, Nalesnik MA, et al. Epstein-Barr virus-induced post-transplant lymphoproliferative disorders: ASTS/ASTP EBV-PTLD Task Force and The Mayo Clinic Organized International Consensus Development Meeting. *Transplantation*. 1999;68:1517–1525.
7. Maruyama D, Watanabe T, Beppu Y, et al. Primary bone lymphoma: A new and detailed characterization of 28 patients in a single-institution study. *Jpn J Clin Oncol*. 2007;37(3):216–223.
8. Leval L, Braaten KM, Ancukiewicz M, et al. Diffuse large B-cell lymphoma of bone. An analysis of differentiation-associated antigens with clinical correlation. *Am J Surg Pathol*. 2003;27:1269–1277.
9. Krishnan A, Shirkhoda A, Tehranzadeh J, Armin AR, Irwin R, Les K. Primary bone lymphoma: Radiographic-MR imaging correlation. *RadioGraphics*. 2003;23:1371–1383.
10. de Camargo PO, Machado TMS, Croci AT, et al. Primary bone lymphoma in 24 patients treated between 1955 and 1999. *Clin Orthop*. 2002;397:271–280.
11. Ramadan KM, Shenkier T, Sehn LH, et al. A clinicopathological retrospective study of 131 patients with primary bone lymphoma: A population-based study of successively treated cohorts from the British Columbia Cancer Agency. *Ann Oncol*. 2007;18:129.
12. Ostrowski ML, Unni KK, Banks PM, et al. Malignant lymphoma of bone. *Cancer*. 1986;58:2646–2655.

CHAPTER 19

A DIAGNOSIS OF EXCLUSION

IRIS O. YUNG
Department of Medicine, California Pacific Medical Center, San Francisco, California

THOMAS E. BAUDENDISTEL
Department of Medicine, Kaiser Permanente Medical Center, Oakland, California

GURPREET DHALIWAL
Department of Medicine, University of California, San Francisco, California; Medical Service, San Francisco VA Medical Center, San Francisco, California

A 26-year-old woman was brought to the emergency department (ED) following new onset of seizures. The patient's friend witnessed several 15-minute episodes of sudden jerks and tremors of her right arm during which the patient bit her tongue, had word-finding difficulty, had horizontal eye deviation, and was incontinent of urine. She became unresponsive during the episodes, with incomplete recovery of consciousness between attacks. She was afebrile. Her neurologic exam 4 hours after several seizures revealed word-finding difficulty and right arm weakness. A complete blood count, chemistry panel including renal and liver function tests, urine toxicology screen, and computed tomography (CT) of the head were normal. After a loading dose of fosphenytoin, the patient did not experience further seizures and was discharged on a maintenance dose of phenytoin.

Over the next week, the patient continued to note a sensation of heaviness in her right arm and felt fatigued. The patient's mother brought her back to the ED after witnessing a similar seizure episode that persisted for an hour. On arrival, the patient was no longer seizing.

Although it can sometimes be difficult to differentiate between seizure, stroke, syncope, and other causes of transient loss of consciousness, this constellation of symptoms strongly points to a seizure. I would classify the patient's focal arm movements associated with impaired consciousness as partial complex seizures. One of the first considerations is determining whether the seizure is caused by a systemic process or by an intrinsic central nervous system (CNS) disorder. Common systemic illnesses include infections, metabolic disturbances, toxins, and malignancies, none of which is evident on the preliminary evaluation. The absence of fever is important as is the time frame (now extending over 1 week) in excluding acute bacterial meningitis. A negative urine toxicology is very helpful but does not exclude the possibility that the seizure is from unmeasured drug intoxication, for example, tricyclic antidepressants, or from drug withdrawal, for example, benzodiazepines, barbiturates, ethanol, and antiepileptic drugs. The persistent right arm heaviness and right arm jerking during the seizures suggest a left cortical focus

Clinical Care Conundrums: Challenging Diagnoses in Hospital Medicine, First Edition.
Edited by James C. Pile, Thomas E. Baudendistel, and Brian J. Harte.

that the CT scan did not detect. Without a clear diagnosis and with recurrent seizures despite antiepileptic drugs, hospitalization is warranted.

The patient experienced migraine headaches each month during menses. There was no family history of seizures. Her only medication was phenytoin. The mother was unaware of any use of tobacco, alcohol, or recreational drugs. The patient was raised in New Jersey and moved to the San Francisco Bay area 9 months previously. She had no pets and had traveled to Florida and Montreal in the past 6 months. She was a graduate student in performing arts. During the preceding 2 weeks, she had been under significant stress and had not slept much in preparation for an upcoming production. The patient's mother was not aware of any head trauma, recent illness, fevers, chills, weight loss, photosensitivity, arthralgias, nausea, vomiting, or diarrhea.

Recent sleep deprivation could provoke seizures in a patient with a latent anatomic focus or metabolic predisposition. Nonadherence to antiepileptic drug therapy is the most common reason for patients to present to the ED with seizures; therefore, I would check a phenytoin level to assess whether she is at a therapeutic level and would consider administering another loading dose. In the absence of immunocompromise or unusual activities or exposures, North American travel does not bring to mind additional etiologies.

On exam, temperature was 37.3°C, blood pressure was 148/84 mm Hg, heart rate was 120 per minute, and respiratory rate was 16 per minute. The patient was stuporous and withdrew from painful stimuli. She was unable to speak. Pupils were 4 mm in diameter and reactive to light. No gaze preference or nystagmus was present. There was no meningismus. Deep tendon reflexes were 1+ and symmetrical in both upper and lower extremities. Plantar reflexes were extensor bilaterally. The tone in the right upper extremity was mildly increased compared to the left. The patient demonstrated semipurposeful movement of the limbs, such as reaching for the bed rails with her arms. Examination of the heart, lungs, abdomen, skin, and oropharynx was normal.

The white blood cell count was 22,300/mm^3 with 50% neutrophils, 40% lymphocytes, 7% monocytes, and 3% eosinophils. Results of the chemistry panel including electrolytes, glucose, creatinine, and liver enzymes, urinalysis, and thyroid-stimulating hormone were normal. Serum phenytoin level was 8.1 μg/mL. Urine toxicology screen, obtained after the patient had received lorazepam, was positive only for benzodiazepines. A chest radiograph was normal.

The cerebrospinal fluid (CSF) was colorless, containing 35 white blood cells/mm^3 (48% lymphocytes, 30% neutrophils, 22% monocytes), 3 red blood cells/mm^3, 62 mg/dL protein, and 50 mg/dL glucose. There was no xanthochromia. The CSF was negative for cryptococcal antigen, antibodies to West Nile virus, polymerase chain reaction (PCR) for herpes simplex viruses 1 and 2, and PCR for *Borrelia burgdorferi*. CSF bacterial culture, cryptococcal antigen, and AFB stain were negative. The serum antinuclear antibody (ANA), rheumatoid factor, and rapid plasma reagin were negative. Serum antibodies to human immunodeficiency virus (HIV), hepatitis B and C viruses, B. burgdorferi, and herpes simplex viruses were negative. The erythrocyte sedimentation rate was 25 mm/hour. There was no growth in her blood cultures.

These CSF findings have to be interpreted in light of her clinical picture, as they are congruent with both an aseptic meningitis and encephalitis. In practice, these can be hard to distinguish, but the early and dominant cortical findings (focal neurologic deficits, prominent altered mental status, bilateral extensor plantar reflexes) and absence of meningeal signs favor encephalitis. This CSF profile can be seen in a variety of disease processes causing meningoencephalitis, including partially treated bacterial meningitis; meningitis due to viruses, fungi, mycobacteria, or atypical bacteria (e.g., *Listeria*); neurosarcoidosis; carcinomatous meningitis; and infection or inflammation from a parameningeal focus in the sinuses, epidural space, or brain parenchyma. The negative HIV test limits the list of opportunistic pathogens. The negative ANA substantially lowers the likelihood of systemic lupus erythematosus, an important consideration in a young woman with an inflammatory disorder involving the CNS. Seizure itself can lead to a postictal pleocytosis in the CSF, although this degree of inflammation would be unusual.

Magnetic resonance imaging (MRI) of the brain showed cortical T2 prolongation with significant enhancement with gadolinium in the cortex and leptomeninges of the left parietal and posterotemporal lobes and right cingulate gyrus region (Fig. 19.1). The patient was admitted to the intensive care unit, and phenytoin and levetiracetam were administered. Over the next several days, she remained afebrile, and her leukocytosis resolved. She continued to have seizures every day despite receiving phenytoin and levetiracetam, and adding lamotrigine. She was alert and complained about persistent right arm weakness and word-finding difficulties. Posterior cervical lymphadenopathy at the base of her left occiput was detected on subsequent exam.

An excisional lymph node biopsy demonstrated extensive necrosis without evidence of granulomata, malignancy, or lymphoproliferative disease. Stains and cultures for bacteria, fungi, and mycobacteria were negative. The patient's electroencephalogram captured epileptiform activity over the left hemisphere 2 hours after a cluster of seizures. Brain MR angiography (MRA) and cerebral angiography demonstrated no abnormalities.

Despite this additional information, there is no distinguishing clue that points to a single diagnosis. This is a 26-year-old healthy, seemingly immunocompetent woman who has had a 2-week progressive and refractory seizure disorder secondary to a multifocal neuroinvasive process with a CSF pleocytosis. She does not have evidence of a systemic underlying disorder, save for nonspecific localized lymphadenopathy and a transient episode of leukocytosis on admission, and has no distinguishing epidemiological factors or exposures.

Despite my initial concerns for infectious meningoencephalitis, the negative stains, serologies, and cultures of the blood, CSF, and lymph nodes in the setting of a

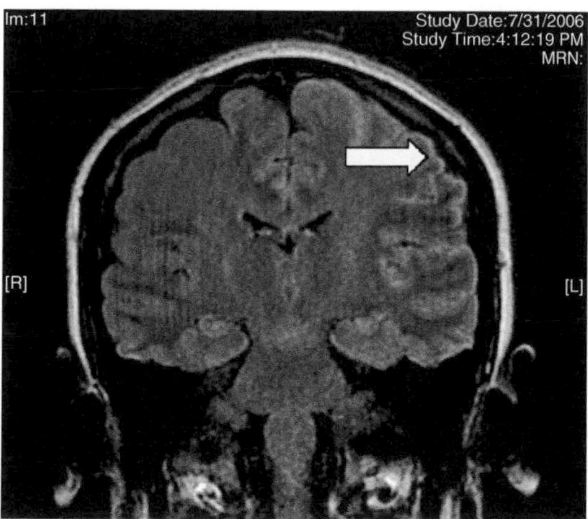

FIGURE 19.1 Brain MRI showed high-intensity FLAIR foci in the cortex and leptomeninges of left parietal (arrow) and posterotemporal lobes and right cingulate gyrus region.

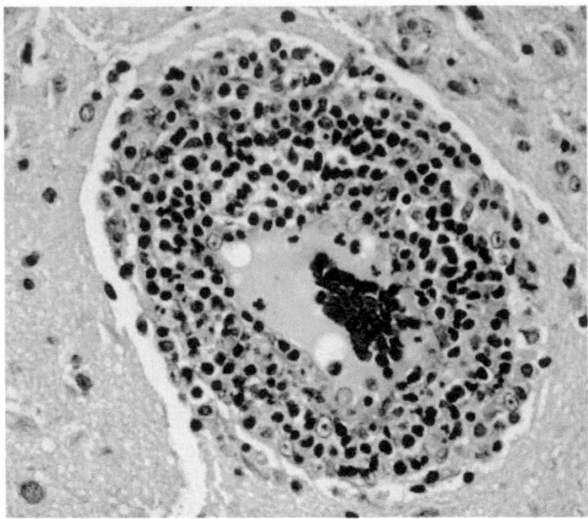

FIGURE 19.2 Biopsy of the leptomeninges and cortex of the left parietal lobe showed multiple blood vessels infiltrated by lymphocytes, neutrophils, and eosinophils consistent with PACNS.

normal immune system and no suspect exposure substantially lower this probability. Arthropod-borne viruses are still possible, especially West Nile virus, because the serological tests are less sensitive early in the illness, acknowledging that the absence of fever, weakness, and known mosquito bites detracts from this diagnosis. Pathogens that cause regional lymphadenopathy and encephalitis, such as *Bartonella*, remain possibilities, as the history of exposure to a kitten can be easily overlooked.

Rheumatologic disorders merit close attention in a young woman, but the negative ANA makes lupus cerebritis unlikely, and the two angiograms did not detect evidence of vasculitis. Finally, there is the question of malignancy and other miscellaneous infiltrative disorders (such as sarcoid), which are of importance here because of the multifocal cortical involvement on imaging.

At this point, I would resample the CSF for viral etiologies (e.g., West Nile virus) and cytology and would send serum *Bartonella* serologies. If these studies were negative, a brain biopsy, primarily to exclude malignancy and also to uncover an unsuspected process, would be indicated. I cannot make a definitive diagnosis or find a perfect fit here, but in the absence of strong evidence of an infection, I am concerned about a malignancy, perhaps a low-grade primary brain tumor.

Brain biopsy of the leptomeninges and cortex of the left parietal lobe showed multiple blood vessels infiltrated by lymphocytes, neutrophils, and eosinophils (Fig. 19.2). The pattern of inflammation was consistent with primary angiitis of the central nervous system (PACNS). The patient received 1 g of intravenous methylprednisolone on three consecutive days, followed by oral prednisone and cyclophosphamide. The seizures ceased, and she made steady progress with rehabilitation therapy. Four months after discharge, a cerebral angiogram (done to ensure there was no interval evidence of vasculitis prior to tapering therapy) demonstrated patency of all major intracranial arteries and venous sinuses.

COMMENTARY

When a patient presents with symptoms or signs referable to the CNS, one must simultaneously consider primary neurologic disorders and systemic diseases that involve the

CNS. Initial evaluation includes a thorough history and physical examination, basic lab studies, routine CSF analysis, and neuroimaging (often a CT scan of the head). Complicated neurologic cases may warrant more elaborate testing including EEG, brain MRI, cerebral angiography, and specialized blood and CSF studies. Clinicians may still find themselves faced with a patient who has clear CNS dysfunction but no obvious diagnosis despite an exhaustive and expensive evaluation. Several disorders match this profile, including intravascular lymphoma, prion diseases, paraneoplastic syndromes, and cerebritis. PACNS, a rare disorder characterized by inflammation of the medium-sized and small arteries of the CNS, is among these disorders. Although the aforementioned diseases sometimes have suggestive or even pathognomonic features (e.g., the "string of beads" angiographic appearance in vasculitides), they are challenging to diagnose when such findings are absent.

Like any vasculitis of the CNS, PACNS may present with a wide spectrum of clinical features.[1,2] Although headache and altered mental status are the most common complaints, paresis, seizures, ataxia, visual changes, and aphasia have all been described. The onset of symptoms ranges from acute to chronic, and neurologic deficits can be focal or diffuse. Systemic manifestations such as fever and weight loss are rare. The average age of onset is 42 years, with no significant sex preponderance. The histopathology of PACNS is granulomatous inflammation of arteries in the parenchyma and leptomeninges of the brain and less commonly in the spinal cord. The narrowing of the affected vessels causes cerebral ischemia and the associated neurologic deficits. The trigger for this focal inflammation is unknown.

After common disorders have been excluded in cases of CNS dysfunction, compatible CSF findings and imaging results may prompt consideration of PACNS. CSF analysis in patients with PACNS typically demonstrates a lymphocytic pleocytosis. Brain MRI abnormalities in PACNS include multiple infarcts in the cortex, deep white matter, or leptomeninges.[3,4] Less specific findings are contrast enhancement in the leptomeninges and white matter disease, both of which may direct the site for meningeal and brain biopsy.

Both brain MRA and cerebral angiography have a limited role in the diagnosis of vasculitis within the CNS. In 18 patients with CNS vasculitis due to autoimmune disease, all had parenchymal abnormalities on MRA but only 65% had evidence of vasculitis on angiography. In two retrospective studies of patients with suspected PACNS, abnormal angiograms had a specificity less than 30% for PACNS, whereas brain biopsies had a negative predictive value of 70%.[5–7] Although in practice, patients with compatible clinical features are sometimes diagnosed with CNS vasculitis on the basis of angiographic findings, brain biopsy is necessary to differentiate vasculitis from other vasculopathies and to establish a definitive diagnosis.

Before a diagnosis of PACNS is made, care must be taken to exclude infections, neoplasms, and autoimmune processes that cause angiitis of the CNS (Table 19.1). The presence of any extracranial abnormalities (which were not present in this case) should prompt consideration of an underlying systemic disorder causing a secondary CNS vasculitis and should cast doubt on the diagnosis of PACNS. Meningovascular syphilis and tuberculosis are among the long list of infections that may cause inflammation of the CNS vasculature. Autoimmune disorders that may cause vasculitis inside the brain include polyarteritis nodosa and Wegener's granulomatosis. Reversible cerebral vasoconstrictive disease, which is most commonly seen in women aged 20–50 years, and sympathomimetic toxins such as cocaine and amphetamine may exhibit clinical and angiographic abnormalities indistinguishable from PACNS.[8,9]

TABLE 19.1 Systemic Diseases that Cause CNS Vasculopathy

Infection: Viruses (HIV varicella-zoster virus, hepatitis C virus), syphilis, *Borrelia burgdorferi*, *Bartonella*, *Mycobacterium tuberculosis*, fungi (*Aspergillus*, *Coccidioides*), bacteria
Autoimmune disorder: Polyarteritis nodosa, Wegener's granulomatosis, temporal arteritis, cryoglobulinemic vasculitis, lupus vasculitis, rheumatoid vasculitis
Toxins: Amphetamine, cocaine, ephedrine, heroin
Malignancy: Primary CNS lymphoma, angioimmunoproliferative disorders, infiltrating glioma

There are no prospective trials investigating PACNS treatment. Aggressive immunosuppression with cyclophosphamide and glucocorticoids is the mainstay of treatment. The duration of treatment varies with the severity of the disease and response to therapy. One study suggests that treatment should be continued for 6–12 months.[10] Neurologic deficits may remain irreversible because of scarring of the affected vessels. Serial brain MRI examinations are often used to follow radiographic resolution during and after the therapy, although radiographic changes do not predict clinical response.[11] New abnormalities on MRI, however, delay any tapering of treatment. The availability of neuroimaging studies and immunosuppressive therapy has improved the prognosis of PACNS. One study reported a favorable outcome with a 29% relapse rate and a 10% mortality rate in 54 patients over a mean follow-up period of 35 months.[12]

PACNS remains a challenging diagnosis because of its rarity, the wide range of neurologic manifestations, and the difficulty in establishing a diagnosis noninvasively. It is an extremely uncommon disease but should be considered in patients with unexplained neurologic deficits referable to the CNS alone after an exhaustive workup. Ultimately, the diagnosis is made by a thorough history and physical examination, exclusion of underlying conditions (particularly systemic vasculitides and infections), and histological confirmation.

Key Points

1. Serious disorders that may present with CNS abnormalities and nondiagnostic abnormal findings on lumbar puncture, brain MRI, and cerebral angiography include intravascular lymphoma, prion diseases, cerebritis, paraneoplastic syndromes, and CNS vasculitis.
2. PACNS is a challenging diagnosis with varied clinical features and often normal angiographic findings. In particular, the specificity of brain MRA and cerebral angiography is low. Although PACNS is rare, it should be on the differential diagnosis in patients with unexplained neurologic deficits referable to the CNS alone, as the condition is fatal without prompt treatment.
3. A diagnosis of PACNS is made only after excluding secondary causes of CNS vasculitis such as infections, malignancies, autoimmune conditions, reversible cerebral vasoconstrictive disease, and medications. The diagnosis is confirmed with a biopsy of the brain and meninges.

REFERENCES

1. Jennette JC, Falk RJ. Medical progress: Small-vessel vasculitis. *N Engl J Med*. 1997;337:1512–1523.
2. Koopman WJ, Moreland LW. *Arthritis and allied conditions: A textbook of rheumatology*. 15th ed. Philadelphia: Lippincott Williams & Wilkins; 2005.

3. Shoemaker EI, Lin ZS, Rae-Grant AD, Little B. Primary angiitis of the central nervous system: Unusual MR appearance. *Am J Neuroradiol*. 1994;15:331–334.
4. Wynne PJ, Younger DS, Khandji A, Silver AJ. Radiographic features of central nervous system vasculitis. *Neurol Clin*. 1997;15:779–804.
5. Kadkhodayan Y, Alreshaid A, Moran CJ, Cross DT 3rd, Powers WJ, Derdeyn CP. Primary angiitis of the central nervous system at conventional angiography. *Radiology*. 2004;233:878–882.
6. Pomper MG, Miller TJ, Stone JH, Tidmore WC, Hellmann DB. CNS vasculitis in autoimmune disease: MR imaging findings and correlation with angiography. *Am J Neuroradiol*. 1999;20:75–85.
7. Duna GF, Calabrese LH. Limitations of invasive modalities in the diagnosis of primary angiitis of the central nervous system. *J Rheumatol*. 1995;22:662–667.
8. Buxton N, McConachie NS. Amphetamine abuse and intracranial haemorrhage. *J R Soc Med*. 2000;93:472–477.
9. Calabrese LH, Duna GF. Drug-induced vasculitis. *Curr Opin Rheumatol*. 1996;8:34–40.
10. Calabrese LH, Duna GF, Lie JT. Vasculitis in the central nervous system. *Arthritis Rheum*. 1997;40:1189–1201.
11. Calabrese LH. Therapy of systemic vasculitis. *Neurol Clin*. 1997;15:973–991.
12. Hajj-Ali RA, Villa-Forte A, Abou-Chebel A, et al. Long-term outcomes of patients with primary angiitis of the central nervous system. *Arthritis Rheum*. 2000;43:S162.

CHAPTER **20**

MAKING A LIST AND CHECKING IT TWICE

SATYEN NICHANI
Division of General Medicine, Department of Internal Medicine, University of Michigan, Ann Arbor, Michigan

SANDRO CINTI
Division of Infectious Diseases, Department of Internal Medicine, University of Michigan, Ann Arbor, Michigan

JEFFREY H. BARSUK
Division of Hospital Medicine, Department of Medicine, Northwestern University Feinberg School of Medicine, Chicago, Illinois

In October, a 36-year-old woman with no significant past medical history presented to the emergency department (ED) with a 3-day history of headache and fever. The headache was severe, throbbing, and frontal in location. She also complained of daily fevers measured up to 103°F, generalized malaise, and fatigue. She did not report neck stiffness or photophobia. She felt better after receiving intravenous fluids and was discharged home with a diagnosis of a nonspecific viral illness. Two days later, she returned to the ED with worsening headache, fever, mild photophobia, and poor oral intake. She also complained of a dry cough that made her headache worse, as did bending over. She did not report confusion, neck stiffness, shortness of breath, sore throat, runny nose, abdominal symptoms, or rash.

This patient presents a second time to the ED with worsening headache and fever, raising concerns about meningitis. At the time of her first ED visit, it can be assumed that she had a nontoxic appearance because she was discharged shortly thereafter. Thus, acute bacterial meningitis seems less likely, but occasionally patients with meningococcal meningitis may not appear significantly ill until later in the process. Nonetheless, acute meningitis, possibly viral, is the initial concern. The time of the year is an important variable because many viral infections are seasonal. Enteroviruses are the most common cause of viral meningitis in the United States, particularly in the summer and fall. In contrast, mumps, measles, and varicella zoster viruses occur more commonly in winter and spring. Herpetic meningoencephalitis is a life-threatening condition with a guarded prognosis. Therefore, early recognition and treatment is necessary to decrease morbidity and mortality. Drugs such as nonsteroidal anti-inflammatory agents, trimethoprim-sulfamethoxazole, amoxicillin, and rarely vaccines can also cause aseptic meningitis. Infections from fungi, spirochetes, mycobacteria, and rarely parasites also cause meningitis, but would be of

Clinical Care Conundrums: Challenging Diagnoses in Hospital Medicine, First Edition.
Edited by James C. Pile, Thomas E. Baudendistel, and Brian J. Harte.

greater concern in a patient with risk factors such as recent travel or an immunocompromised state.

In addition to routine initial tests, cerebrospinal fluid (CSF) analysis and human immunodeficiency virus (HIV) testing are appropriate.

Her past medical history was notable for depression. Her medications included bupropion, multivitamins, and fish oil. She was also taking milk thistle pills daily to "protect her liver" because she had been drinking alcohol heavily for the past 2 weeks since her husband left her. She smoked 1 pack of cigarettes daily. She had not traveled recently. She reported no recent animal or wildlife exposure but did recall falling into a Midwestern river while canoeing 2 weeks prior to presentation. She worked as a hairstylist and described no sick contacts or risk factors for HIV.

If she swallowed a significant amount of water during her fall overboard, meningitis from waterborne infections such as *Aeromonas, Acanthamoeba*, and *Naegleria* need to be considered. Fortunately, these are rare in the Midwest. Her canoeing history may also suggest exposure to wooded areas, and tick-borne infections such as ehrlichiosis, babesiosis, Lyme disease, and Rocky Mountain spotted fever can also cause meningitis. Histoplasmosis and blastomycosis are also endemic to the midwestern United States and can disseminate and cause central nervous system disease.

At this time, viral and bacterial infections are highest on the differential diagnosis. However, the microbiology laboratory needs to be alerted on the possibility of fungal or parasitic organisms depending on the initial CSF analysis results.

The patient was a Caucasian woman who appeared comfortable. Her blood pressure was 130/62 mm Hg, heart rate was 83 beats per minute, respiratory rate was 18 per minute, temperature was 100.8°F, and oxygen saturation was 98% on room air. She was fully alert and oriented. Her pupils were bilaterally equal, reactive to light and accommodation with intact extraocular movement and no nystagmus. There was conjunctival injection bilaterally without noticeable pallor or icterus. Fundoscopic examination, which the patient tolerated without difficulty, was normal. Inspection of the oral cavity showed mild tonsillar enlargement. The neck was supple with no stiffness. No cervical, axillary, or inguinal lymph nodes were palpable. Faint bilateral basilar crackles were audible over the posterior chest. There was very mild right upper quadrant abdominal tenderness without guarding. The liver and spleen were normal in size and bowel sounds were present. No rash, peripheral edema, or spinal tenderness was noted. A complete neurological examination was normal.

Her general appearance and vital signs are reassuring. Conjunctival injection and mild tonsillar enlargement are nonspecific findings and may occur in systemic inflammatory states especially viral infections. Atelectasis may account for faint bilateral basilar crackles, especially if associated with post-tussive change. Her alcohol use puts her at risk of aspiration. A right lower lobe process (pneumonia) can sometimes present with right upper quadrant tenderness. However, this tenderness may also represent muscle soreness from repeated coughing, liver, or gallbladder disease. The same infectious process affecting the central nervous system and possibly her lungs may also be affecting the liver.

A complete blood count revealed a white blood cell count of 3000/mm^3 (79% neutrophils, 15% lymphocytes, 5% monocytes), hemoglobin of 11.7 g/dL, and platelets of 110,000/mm^3. The serum sodium was 133 mmol/L, potassium was 3.7 mmol/L, bicarbonate was 22 mmol/L, and blood urea nitrogen was 20 mg/dL. The serum creatinine was 1.5 compared to 1.0 mg/dL on testing 2 days prior.

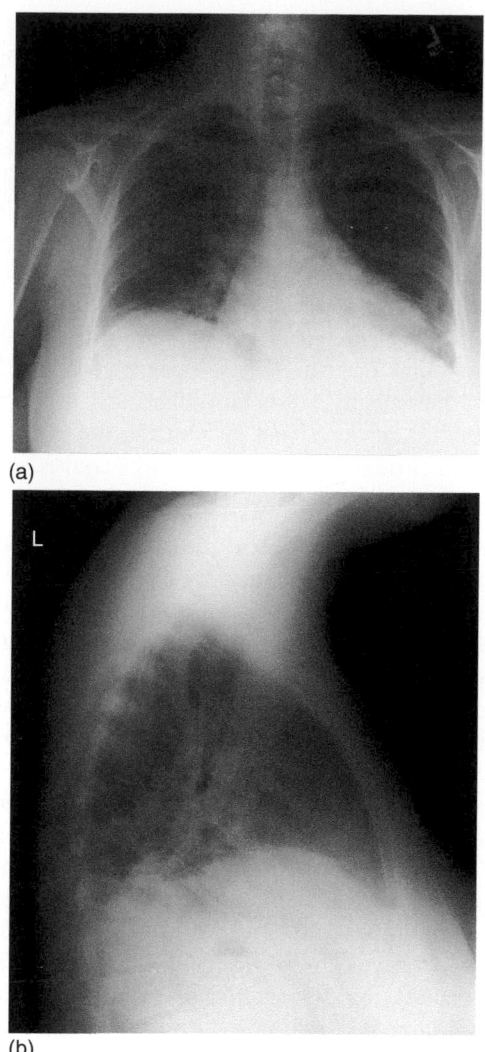

FIGURE 20.1 Admission chest X-ray: (a) posteroanterior and (b) lateral views.

A liver function panel showed protein of 5.1 g/dL, albumin of 3 g/dL, aspartate aminotransferase (AST) of 576 IU/L, alanine aminotransferase (ALT) of 584 IU/L, alkaline phosphatase of 282 IU/L, and total bilirubin of 1 mg/dL. The coagulation profile, creatinine phosphokinase, acetaminophen level, urine pregnancy test, urine drug screen, and urinalysis (including urine microscopy) were normal.

The CSF opening pressure was 13 cm H_2O. CSF analysis showed four mononuclear leukocytes per high-power field, CSF protein was 27 mg/dL, and glucose was 76 mg/dL. No organisms were noted on Gram stain. A chest X-ray showed focal airspace opacity in the left lower lobe (Fig. 20.1), and the patient was hospitalized for further management.

The normal CSF analysis makes acute meningitis much less likely. It is interesting to note that the aminotransferase levels are nearly equal. In viral and many other causes of hepatitis, the ALT is usually higher than the AST, whereas the contrary is true in alcoholic hepatitis. Because the patient has been consuming significant amounts of alcohol recently, these levels may become equal in the setting of another underlying liver process. The elevation in liver enzymes also raises the possibility of autoimmune hepatitis secondary to a systemic vasculitis such as systemic lupus erythematosus. Nonetheless, the focus should be on infectious causes of hepatitis such as hepatitis C, adenovirus, parvovirus, Epstein-Barr virus (EBV), cytomegalovirus, and herpes simplex virus that can cause pneumonia as either a primary or a secondary infection. Acute HIV infection can also present in this fashion, and anti-HIV antibody testing may be negative early in the disease. In the setting of a normal urinalysis and bland urine sediment, prerenal azotemia is the most likely cause of her acute renal injury and can be confirmed by testing the urinary sodium and creatinine. A peripheral smear should be reviewed to evaluate pancytopenia.

Severe headache, fever, conjunctival injection, pancytopenia, acute kidney injury, hepatitis, and pneumonia may occur in leptospirosis, particularly in a patient with recent freshwater exposure. Alternatively, ehrlichiosis can also account for fever, headache, pancytopenia, renal failure, hepatitis, and pneumonia, but conjunctival suffusion is not often present. At this time, treatment for community-acquired pneumonia that includes coverage for leptospirosis should be started.

The patient was hydrated with intravenous fluids and treated with intravenous ceftriaxone and azithromycin for community-acquired pneumonia. An abdominal ultrasound was normal. The serologic assays for acute hepatitis A, B, and C infection were negative. The following morning, she reported worsening headache, increased cough now productive of whitish yellow sputum, and diffuse body aches. She appeared more lethargic and toxic. Her blood pressure was 100/83 mm Hg, heart rate was 84 beats per minute, respiratory rate was 24 per minute, and temperature was 101.3°F. She had increased crackles on chest auscultation bilaterally and required supplemental oxygen at 4 L per minute by nasal cannula. Examination of both legs now revealed multiple scattered, faintly erythematous, 2-cm-sized patches overlying tender subtle subcutaneous nodules. Additionally, a mildly pruritic, V-shaped area of blanchable erythema was also seen on her chest. The white blood cell count was 2500/mm^3 (77% neutrophils, 15% lymphocytes), serum creatinine was 1.8 mg/dL, AST was 351 IU/L, and ALT was 485 IU/L. Blood cultures showed no growth and a peripheral smear examination was unrevealing. A noncontrast chest computed tomographic scan showed findings consistent with multifocal pneumonia (Fig. 20.2).

It would be prudent at this time to expand her antimicrobial coverage for activity against methicillin-resistant *Staphylococcus aureus* and *Pseudomonas*. Although

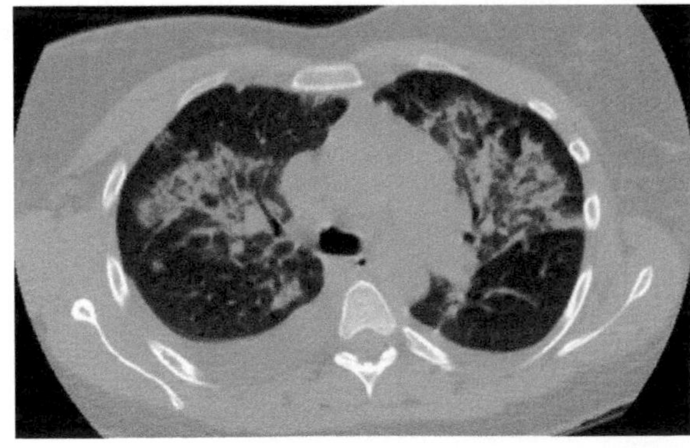

FIGURE 20.2 Bilateral patchy airspace disease and pleural effusions on chest computed tomographic scan.

ceftriaxone or piperacillin would cover leptospirosis, given the possibility of ehrlichiosis, the addition of doxycycline should be strongly considered.

The description of the rash on her legs seems consistent with erythema nodosum, which is associated with a number of infections (streptococcal, fungal, syphilis, EBV, cat scratch disease, tuberculosis), inflammatory conditions (inflammatory bowel disease, autoimmune disease, malignancy), and pregnancy. The blanchable rash on the chest is also a cause of concern for a possible drug reaction (ceftriaxone). A Jarisch–Herxheimer reaction is possible given her acute worsening of symptoms with initiation of antibiotic therapy.

An antineutrophil cytoplasmic antibody-associated vasculitis or another autoimmune condition such as systemic lupus erythematosus can account for erythema nodosum, rash, pancytopenia, and hepatitis. This diagnosis might also fit if she had a vasculitic pulmonary hemorrhage that caused her lung infiltrates and worsening hypoxia. A complete antinuclear antibody panel, antineutrophil cytoplasmic antibody, and anti-smooth-muscle-antibody testing is recommended. A skin and bronchoscopic biopsy should be considered.

Her dose of ceftriaxone was increased for possible severe pneumococcal pneumonia. The dermatology consultant felt that her leg lesions were consistent with erythema nodosum and the chest rash was consistent with cutaneous photodamage. Bronchoscopic examination was normal and a bronchoalveolar lavage sample showed 2905 red blood cells/mm^3 and 605 white blood cells/mm^3 (70% neutrophils, 7% lymphocytes, 16% histiocytes), normal cytology, and negative cultures. There was no significant clinical improvement by the fourth hospital day and oral doxycycline was started. The next day, her skin lesions had resolved and she felt better. The serologic tests for *Legionella*, *Mycoplasma*, cytomegalovirus, EBV, *Toxoplasma*, *Chlamydophila*, *Ehrlichia*, *Leptospira*, Q fever, parvovirus, and adenovirus were negative. A fungal serology panel, HIV polymerase chain reaction, cryoglobulin level, and several rheumatologic tests (antinuclear antibody, extractable nuclear antigen panel, rheumatoid factor, antineutrophil cytoplasmic antibody, anti-proteinase 3, and anti-glomerular basement membrane antibodies) were normal. Blood cultures continued to show no growth.

The apparent response to doxycycline suggests that she might have ehrlichiosis. A buffy coat review for morulae should be done. It is also possible that she may have improved on her initial therapy alone before starting doxycycline and her clinical worsening (including the chest rash) was due to a Jarisch–Herxheimer reaction. Serologic tests for leptospirosis and ehrlichiosis should be repeated in 1–2 weeks because such infections may not cause detectable antibody levels early in the illness.

Ceftriaxone and doxycycline were continued and she showed rapid and significant clinical improvement. She was discharged 4 days later with instructions to complete a 10-day course of antibiotics. At her 3-month follow-up, she was doing well and a repeat *Leptospira* antibody test by the Indirect Hemagglutination Assay (MRL Diagnostics, Cypress, California; normal titer <1:50) was positive at a titer of 1:100, which is highly suggestive of leptospirosis.

COMMENTARY

Leptospirosis is a zoonotic infection caused by spirochetes of the genus *Leptospira*. The infection is usually transmitted indirectly to humans through contact with water, food, or soil contaminated with the urine of infected mammals.[1] Risk factors for infection

TABLE 20.1 Clinical Manifestations of Leptospirosis[1,4,5]

1. Mild influenza-like self-remitting disease (90% of cases)
   - Undifferentiated *fever* (usually 100–105°F), severe *headache*, and *myalgia* (especially lower limbs).
2. Moderately severe disease usually requiring hospitalization (5%–9% of cases)
   - Marked prostration, anorexia, nausea, and vomiting, *conjunctival suffusion*, *transient rash*, frequent abdominal pain, constipation or diarrhea, and occasionally epistaxis.
3. Severe disease involving multiple organ systems (1%–5% of cases)
   - *Hepatorenal Syndrome (Weil's syndrome)*

   Constellation of jaundice, hemorrhagic diathesis, and *acute renal failure*. Hepatic failure is rarely fatal. Renal involvement is usually more severe and the common cause of death. Cardiac (myocarditis with arrhythmias) and *pulmonary complications* are frequent. Confusion and restlessness may occur.
   - Hemorrhagic pneumonitis

   Usually presents as a dry cough initially but becomes blood-streaked after 2–3 days. Often characterized by a rapid progression to involve extensive areas of lungs, massive intra-alveolar hemorrhage, acute respiratory failure, and death.
   - Central nervous system involvement meningismus, meningitis, or meningoencephalitis.

NOTE: This patient's manifestations are highlighted in italics.

include participation in recreational activities (such as freshwater swimming, canoeing, and camping), occupational exposure, and exposure to infected pets or domesticated livestock. Approximately 100–200 cases are identified annually in the United States, and approximately half occur in the state of Hawaii.[2] Outbreaks of leptospirosis have been reported previously in the Midwest.[3]

These organisms enter humans through contact with mucous membranes or broken skin or by swallowing infected food or water. A large number of these infections remain subclinical or result in a very mild illness with spontaneous clearance by the host's immune mechanism. Following an incubation period of 2–30 days, infected individuals may develop clinically significant disease (Table 20.1). Clinical presentations may overlap as the disease progresses. Although much remains to be learned about the exact pathogenic mechanism, disruption of the cell membranes of small vessel endothelia (a toxin-like effect) and cytokine-mediated tissue injury are believed to cause organ hemorrhage and ischemia.[4]

The clinical diagnosis of leptospirosis is difficult because of its protean manifestations. Although nonspecific, two clinical features may provide a clue to the clinical diagnosis. First, the presence of conjunctival suffusion occurs in the early stage of the disease and is often associated with subconjunctival hemorrhage. Second, severe myalgia, commonly involving the lower limbs, is also characteristically present.[1,5] In a series of 58 patients with acute leptospirosis, conjunctival suffusion was observed in 50% of cases and subconjunctival hemorrhage in 29%. Body ache and muscle tenderness were described in almost all cases.[6]

As seen in this case, the presence of a rash may pose a clinical challenge. A transient macular, maculopapular, purpuric, or urticarial rash may be seen in acute leptospirosis, but rashes may also be representative of a complication of treatment.[1] First described in 1895 in patients with syphilis treated with mercury, the Jarisch–Herxheimer reaction typically occurs within a few hours of antimicrobial treatment of spirochete infections and often presents with a rash, headache, fever, rigors, hypotension, sweating, and worsening symptoms of the underlying illness.[7] Other skin findings, such as the occurrence of erythema nodosum, have been previously reported in cases of leptospirosis.[8]

Human ehrlichiosis (HE) is caused by tick-borne obligatory intracellular bacteria that infect leukocytes. There are three distinct clinical conditions: human monocytic ehrlichiosis (HME, caused by *Ehrlichia chaffeensis*), human granulocytic anaplasmosis (HGA, caused by *Anaplasma phagocytophilum*), and human ewingii ehrlichiosis (HEE, caused by *Ehrlichia ewingii*). Although most cases of HME and HEE are seen in the southeastern and south-central United States and California, the highest incidence of HGA is reported in the northeastern and upper Midwest regions.[9] As with leptospirosis, the clinical range of HE spans from asymptomatic infection to life-threatening illness. Following an incubation period of 1–2 weeks, symptomatic cases usually present with nonspecific complaints such as high fevers, chills, headache, nausea, arthralgia, myalgia, and malaise.[10] The majority of cases will report a tick bite or an exposure to ticks. Laboratory tests often reveal leukopenia (white blood cell count, $<4000/mm^3$), thrombocytopenia, hyponatremia, and elevated AST and ALT. Patients with severe disease may develop renal, respiratory, and hepatic failure. Thus, differentiating ehrlichiosis from leptospirosis is often challenging for the clinician.

However, there are a few clinical clues that help distinguish between these illnesses in this case. HGA as a cause of HE would be more likely in the Midwest. Although a rash is present in one-third of patients with HME, it is seldom present in HGA unless coinfected with *Borrelia burgdorferi*, the causative agent for Lyme disease. Additionally, her history of freshwater exposure and the absence of a history of a tick bite also favor leptospirosis. As noted previously, conjunctival suffusion, a characteristic clinical feature of leptospirosis, has only been described in case reports of HE.[11,12] Although doxycycline is the drug of choice for the treatment of ehrlichiosis, *Leptospira* is susceptible to a wide variety of antibiotics because it exhibits a double membrane surface architecture with components common to both gram-negative and gram-positive bacteria.[1] Recommended treatment regimens for severe leptospirosis include the use of high-dose intravenous penicillin or a third-generation cephalosporin. Less severe cases can be treated with oral amoxicillin or doxycycline.[13]

Serologic tests are often used to establish the diagnosis of leptospirosis and ehrlichiosis. When either condition is on the list of potential diagnoses, a key component of testing is to obtain samples twice in order to catch the acute and convalescent-phase antibodies. Leptospires are fastidious organisms that are difficult to isolate on inoculated growth media. The microscopic agglutination test for leptospirosis is considered the diagnostic gold standard due to its high specificity, but its use is limited by its technical complexity, lack of availability (other than in reference laboratories), and low sensitivity early in the disease (antibody levels detected by this method usually do not appear until 7 days after symptom onset).[14] A variety of rapid serologic assays are also available. Although these tests have good overall sensitivity (ranging between 79% and 93%), they perform relatively poorly for acute-phase sera (sensitivity of 38.5%–52.7%).[14] The high early false-negative rate is believed to be a result of inadequate *Leptospira* antibody titers in the acute phase of the illness. Seroconversion or a four-fold rise between acute- and convalescent-phase antibody titers is the most definitive criterion for the diagnosis of leptospirosis. However, without paired sera samples, a single high microscopic agglutination test titer can be taken as diagnostic for leptospirosis depending on the degree of regional endemicity.[15] Similarly, currently available serologic assays for ehrlichiosis produce negative results in most patients in the first week of illness, and it is important to obtain a convalescent-phase serum specimen for confirmatory diagnosis of HME and HGA.

Seroconversion or a four-fold increase in titer between acute and convalescent-phase sera is considered diagnostic.

Key Points

1. Establishing a diagnosis of leptospirosis is challenging and requires a high index of suspicion. Clinicians should be aware of the limitations of the diagnostic accuracy of the serologic assays for leptospirosis because they are frequently negative in the first week after symptom onset.
2. The classic finding of conjunctival suffusion is helpful in differentiating leptospirosis from HE.
3. This case highlights the importance of the clinical practice of making a list of suspected diagnoses, remaining open to these possibilities, and checking serologic tests again in convalescence to confirm the diagnosis.

Acknowledgments

The authors thank Dr. Brian Harte for his valuable guidance in the preparation of the manuscript.

REFERENCES

1. Vijayachari P, Sugunan AP, Shriram AN. Leptospirosis: An emerging global public health problem. *J Biosci*. 2008;33:557–569.
2. Centers for Disease Control and Prevention. Leptospirosis. 2005. Available at: www.cdc.gov/ncidod/dbmd /diseaseinfo/leptospirosis_t.htm. Accessed November 15, 2010.
3. Morbidity and Mortality Weekly Report. From the Centers for Disease Control and Prevention. Update: leptospirosis and unexplained acute febrile illness among athletes participating in triathlons—Illinois and Wisconsin, 1998. *JAMA*. 1998;280:1474–1475.
4. Pappas G, Cascio A. Optimal treatment of leptospirosis: Queries and projections. *Int J Antimicrob Agents*. 2006;28:491–496.
5. Ricaldi JN, Vinetz JM. Leptospirosis in the tropics and in travelers. *Curr Infect Dis Rep*. 2006;8:51–58.
6. Singh SS, Vijayachari P, Sinha A, Sugunan AP, Rasheed MA, Sehgal SC. Clinico-epidemiological study of hospitalized cases of severe leptospirosis. *Indian J Med Res*. 1999;109:94–99.
7. Pound MW, May DB. Proposed mechanisms and preventative options of Jarisch-Herxheimer reactions. *J Clin Pharm Ther*. 2005;30:291–295.
8. Buckler JM. Leptospirosis presenting with erythema nodosum. *Arch Dis Child*. 1977;52:418–419.
9. Walker DH, Paddock CD, Dumler JS. Emerging and re-emerging tick-transmitted rickettsial and ehrlichial infections. *Med Clin N Am*. 2008;92:1345–1361.
10. Ganguly S, Mukhopadhayay SK. Tick-borne ehrlichiosis infection in human beings. *J Vector Borne Dis*. 2008;45:273–280.
11. Simmons BP, Hughey JR. Ehrlichia in Tennessee. *South Med J*. 1989;82:669.
12. Berry DS, Miller RS, Hooke JA, Massung RF, Bennett J, Ottolini MG. Ehrlichial meningitis with cerebrospinal fluid morulae. *Pediatr Infect Dis J*. 1999;18:552–555.
13. Terpstra WJ, World Health Organization, International Leptospirosis Society. *Human leptospirosis: guidance for diagnosis, surveillance and control*. Geneva, Switzerland: World Health Organization; 2003.
14. Bajani MD, Ashford DA, Bragg SL, et al. Evaluation of four commercially available rapid serologic tests for diagnosis of leptospirosis. *J Clin Microbiol*. 2003;41:803–809.
15. Shivakumar S, Shareek PS. Diagnosis of leptospirosis utilizing modified Faine's criteria. *J Assoc Physicians India*. 2004;52:678–679.

CHAPTER 21

CAUGHT IN THE WEB: E-DIAGNOSIS

YASUHARU TOKUDA

Department of Medicine, Mito Kyodo General Hospital, University of Tsukuba, Mito City, Japan

MAKOTO AOKI

Sakura Seiki Company, Tokyo, Japan

SAURABH B. KANDPAL

Department of Hospital Medicine, Cleveland Clinic, Cleveland, Ohio

LAWRENCE M. TIERNEY JR.

Department of Medicine, University of California, San Francisco, California

A 52-year-old woman presented with a 3-month history of progressive bilateral leg edema and dyspnea while climbing a flight of stairs or while walking up a steep slope. She also complained of a tingling sensation in both hands and fingers, which started about 2 months prior to the onset of edema. She did not describe sensory problems in the lower extremities and did not have any other neurological complaints. She denied fever, cough, chest pain, palpitations, orthopnea, paroxysmal nocturnal dyspnea, and dark stools. She had no history of hypertension, diabetes, dyslipidemia, or asthma and had never been hospitalized. She did not smoke or consume alcohol and used no medications, including over-the-counter drugs or dietary supplements. The patient was born in Japan and had not traveled outside the country since her birth. She was a homemaker and had worked occasionally as a manual laborer in sugarcane agriculture. A review of systems revealed no history of polydipsia, polyuria, or cold or heat intolerance but did identify new hair growth, especially on the extremities.

This middle-aged woman shows progressive changes in her general health status that are characterized by edema and dyspnea on effort. The differential diagnosis of edema includes a broad spectrum of illnesses, such as cardiac, lung, renal, endocrine, and hepatic diseases. Because of the life-threatening potential, my first concern is cardiac disease, although the patient is not experiencing typical symptoms of ischemic heart disease or congestive failure. Bilateral and distal distribution of neuropathic symptoms is likely due to diseases of peripheral nerves rather than those of the central nervous system. Her complaint of a bilateral tingling sensation in the hands may suggest carpal tunnel syndrome as a result of her long-term agricultural work. Other possible causes include radiculopathy of the cervical spine or polyneuropathy. Clues in the physical examination may help narrow the differential diagnosis to a cardiac, hepatic, or endocrine disorder.

Clinical Care Conundrums: Challenging Diagnoses in Hospital Medicine, First Edition.
Edited by James C. Pile, Thomas E. Baudendistel, and Brian J. Harte.

The patient appeared ill. Her weight had increased from 48 to 61 kg since she was last weighed before 6 months. Her blood pressure was 140/78 mm Hg, her heart rate was 72 beats per minute with a regular rhythm, her respiratory rate was 18 per minute, and her temperature was 37.5°C. The jugular venous pressure was elevated at 10 cm above the sternal angle. A grade IMA/I systolic ejection murmur was evident at the second interspace along the left sternal border. The second heart sound was fixed and split. There were decreased breath sounds and complete dullness to percussion over both lower lung fields. Shifting dullness was noted on abdominal examination. There was pitting edema from the feet to the thighs, with slow pit-recovery time in both legs, and she exhibited generalized hirsutism on the face, body, and extremities. There was no lymphadenopathy. On neurological examination, her mental status was normal. The cranial nerves were normal, as was coordination. There was mild generalized distal-dominant motor weakness with generalized hyporeflexia. Sensory testing demonstrated glove-and-stocking type loss of sensation to pinpricks as well as dysesthesia in all extremities. Phalen and Tinel tests were negative.

The elevated venous pressure and pitting edema with slow recovery suggest high venous pressure edema rather than hypoproteinemic edema. Complete bilateral dullness of the chest and shifting dullness of the abdomen indicate the presence of bilateral pleural effusion and ascites. Edema from high venous pressure is usually caused by right, left, or biventricular cardiac failure. A fixed splitting of the second heart sound suggests an atrial septal defect, which is a rare cause of progressive right heart failure in adults. I recommend checking the patient's thyroid function to investigate the possibility of hypothyroidism, which is a common illness among middle-aged women and could contribute to her edema as well as hirsutism. The neurological findings suggest a generalized polyneuropathy. The unusual combination of high venous pressure edema and polyneuropathy may indicate a rare multisystem disorder such as amyloidosis. Alternatively, the patient might have developed multiple diseases during the same time period. For instance, diabetic polyneuropathy is the most common cause of polyneuropathy among the middle-aged. Finally, the differential diagnosis of hirsutism includes ovarian, adrenal, or pituitary sources of hyperandrogenism in addition to hypothyroidism. I would first evaluate for diabetes, thyroid disease, and cardiac disease and would like to see the results of laboratory tests for thyrotropin and plasma glucose, as well as chest radiography and electrocardiography.

The white blood cell count was 5400/mm^3 with a normal differential. Hemoglobin was 10.7 g/dL with normal red-cell indices, and the platelet count was 276,000/mm^3. The erythrocyte sedimentation rate was 29 mm/hour. Other laboratory tests revealed the following values: total protein, 6.2 g/dL; albumin, 3.3 g/dL; blood urea nitrogen, 12 mg/dL; creatinine, 0.7 mg/dL; aspartate aminotransferase, 6 U/L; alanine aminotransferase, 2 U/L; lactate dehydrogenase, 96 U/L; alkaline phosphatase, 115 U/L; creatine phosphokinase, 60 U/L; total bilirubin, 0.9 mg/dL; glucose, 96 mg/dL; hemoglobin A1c, 4.6%; total cholesterol, 111 mg/dL; and thyrotropin, 6.32 mIU/mL (normal range, 0.50–5.00 mIU/mL). Serum free thyroxine, triiodothyronine, and urine testosterone were normal. Serum dehydroepiandrosterone sulfate was mildly elevated for her age (864 ng/mL: normal range, 180–750 ng/mL). Serological studies for human immunodeficiency virus, human T-lymphotrophic virus type 1, and syphilis were negative. Urinalysis was weakly positive for protein but negative for casts and occult blood. The stool was negative for occult blood. A chest radiograph showed bilateral pleural

effusions. Computed tomography demonstrated bilateral pleural effusions, ascites, mild hepatomegaly, and small, multiple, mediastinal lymph nodes. Her electrocardiogram was normal. A transesophageal echocardiogram with agitated saline contrast demonstrated normal ventricular systolic and diastolic function and no atrial septal defect. The inferior vena cava did not collapse with inspiration, and there was no evidence of infiltrative cardiomyopathy.

These laboratory results rule out diabetes as the cause of the polyneuropathy. The subclinical hypothyroidism would not explain profound edema and hirsutism. A serum albumin level of 3.3 g/dL confirms high venous pressure edema rather than hypoproteinemic edema. Normochromic, normocytic anemia and a mildly elevated sedimentation rate point to a chronic illness or an inflammatory state. The mediastinal lymphadenopathy may reflect congestion as a result of the high venous pressure or reflect a systemic disease involving lymph nodes. Normal ventricular function with high venous pressure is suggestive of heart failure from diastolic dysfunction, although the patient does not have risk factors for diastolic dysfunction, such as hypertension, and has no other echocardiographic features of diastolic impairment. The combination of hyperandrogenism and neuropathy point toward a systemic process, such as a paraneoplastic syndrome. I would next investigate the source of the excess androgens.

Because serum dehydroepiandrosterone sulfate was mildly elevated, I-131 aldosterol scintigraphy was performed, and it was negative. Electromyography showed a pattern of generalized sensorimotor polyneuropathy.

At this point, it appears that cardiac, endocrine, hepatic, and renal diseases have been largely ruled out as the cause of her symptoms. Reframing and unifying the important clinical problems for this patient may be useful in resolving this diagnostic puzzle. They include (i) systemic high venous pressure edema; (ii) generalized sensorimotor polyneuropathy; (iii) hirsutism; (iv) normocytic, normochromic anemia; (v) an elevated erythrocyte sedimentation rate; (vi) mediastinal lymphadenopathy; and (vii) subclinical hypothyroidism. At this point, I cannot unify these pieces of information into a single diagnosis. I would search the medical literature, focusing on these terms.

A general internist consultant performed MEDLINE and Google Scholar searches using the key words "edema," "polyneuropathy," and "hirsutism." This search suggested the diagnosis of Crow–Fukase syndrome, also known as POEMS (polyneuropathy, organomegaly, endocrinopathy, M protein, and skin changes) syndrome. Subsequent evaluations were performed. First, serum protein electrophoresis revealed the presence of monoclonal proteins, although hypergammaglobulinemia was not present. Second, bone marrow examination demonstrated increased abnormal plasma cell proliferation (7%), although a radiographic skeletal survey found no lesions suggestive of plasmacytoma. Third, cerebrospinal fluid analysis showed normal cell counts but increased protein concentration (202 mg/dL). Fourth, a blood sample referred to an outside laboratory demonstrated elevated levels of vascular endothelial growth factor (3902 pg/mL: normal range, 150–500 pg/mL). On the basis of these findings, the diagnosis of POEMS syndrome was made. After oral prednisolone (40 mg/day) was initiated, the systemic edema improved gradually, and she did well during the 2-year follow-up period.

COMMENTARY

POEMS syndrome, also known as the *Crow–Fukase syndrome*, is a rare multisystem disorder first described by Crow in 1956.[1,2] It is characterized by polyneuropathy,

TABLE 21.1 Criteria for the Diagnosis of POEMS Syndrome

Major criteria	Polyneuropathy
	Monoclonal plasma cell-proliferative disorder
Minor criteria	Sclerotic bone lesions
	Castleman disease
	Organomegaly (splenomegaly, hepatomegaly, or lymphadenopathy)
	Edema (peripheral edema, pleural effusion, or ascites)
	Endocrinopathy (adrenal, thyroid, pituitary, gonadal, parathyroid, or pancreatic)
	Skin changes (hyperpigmentation, hirsutism, plethora, hemangiomata, and white nails)
	Papilledema

NOTE: Two major criteria and at least one minor criterion are required for diagnosis.
Abbreviation: POEMS, polyneuropathy, organomegaly, endocrinopathy, M protein, and skin changes.
This table is based on the work of Dispenzieri.[7]

organomegaly, endocrinopathy, monoclonal gammopathy, and skin changes, as indicated by the acronym. The diagnosis of POEMS syndrome is difficult, as this syndrome is rare and requires high clinical suspicion. According to a nationwide cross-sectional survey in Japan, the prevalence of POEMS syndrome is very low (about 3 patients per 1,000,000 persons),[3] and its prevalence in the Western countries is considered even lower than that in Japan. The average age at onset is around 45–50 years, and men are twice as likely to have this syndrome as women.[4–6] Table 21.1 shows the diagnostic criteria of POEMS syndrome, based on the research by Dispenzieri and others at the Mayo Clinic, and Table 21.2 presents the relative frequency of these clinical features.[6,7] The initial symptomatology generally includes polyneuropathy, skin changes, and generalized edema, which are nonspecific symptoms, as are other well-recognized associated conditions such as clubbing, weight loss, thrombocytosis, polycythemia, and hyperhidrosis. Thus, it is important to consider this syndrome when one is facing an undiagnosed illness involving multiple organ systems and to distinguish it from other conditions such as multiple myeloma, amyloidosis, and monoclonal gammopathy of undetermined significance. Vascular endothelial growth factor is thought to be involved in the edema of POEMS syndrome, as massive release from aggregated platelets increases vascular permeability and venous pressure.[7–10]

Data regarding treatment and survival are largely observational. Overall mean survival from diagnosis in the 2003 Dispenzieri cohort was 13.7 years, with death often due to infection or cardiorespiratory failure.[6] When a solitary plasmacytoma or osteosclerotic myeloma is present, radiation to the lesion can often lead to clinical remission. Other treatment options include alkylating agents and/or high-dose chemotherapy with peripheral stem cell transplantation, corticosteroids, and supportive care.[7]

Clinicians frequently use the Internet to aid in the clinical decision process. In a survey of the Royal New Zealand College of General Practitioners,[11] half reported that they used the Internet to search for clinical information. Two well-known resources are MEDLINE, which contains over 11 million references dating back to the 1960s, and internet search engines such as Google (and a more recent product, Google Scholar, which attempts to sort search results by including factors such as the author, the publication in which the article appears, and how often the article has been cited).

MEDLINE searches a well-defined set of journals and uses the Medical Subject Headings (MeSH) vocabulary, which consists of sets of descriptive terms organized in a

TABLE 21.2 Relative Frequency of Clinical Features in Patients with POEMS Syndrome ($n = 99$)

Characteristic	%
Peripheral neuropathy	100
Monoclonal plasma cell dyscrasia	100
Sclerotic bone lesions	97
Endocrinopathy	71
Skin changes	68
Organomegaly	46
Extravascular volume overload	39
Papilledema	29
Castleman disease	11

This table is based on the work of Dispenzieri.[7]
Abbreviation: POEMS, polyneuropathy, organomegaly, endocrinopathy, M protein, and skin changes.

hierarchical structure to allow searching with various levels of specificity. For instance, entering the term *heart attack* will map to the MeSH term *myocardial infarction* and will also include more specific terms such as *myocardial stunning* and *cardiogenic shock*.

Google, in comparison, explores resources beyond journals without any clear boundary to its scope, and its advanced search functions can be occasionally unreliable. For instance, search results are occasionally marred by outdated citation information and may include materials that are not truly scholarly. However, search engines can search through the actual text of manuscripts and access the "gray literature," which includes open-source material that is usually original but not widely distributed or often easily available, such as technical reports and dissertations. A direct study comparing the results of searches in PubMed (one of the MEDLINE search engines) and Google Scholar is difficult, but the critical characteristics of each can be compared and contrasted (Table 21.3).

Internet searches may also suggest diagnoses from a compilation of clinical features, such as in this case. To be successful, such a search must complement the cognitive process; a search engine cannot completely replace clinical judgment. Clinicians must be able to identify salient clinical features and generate high-yield search terms and then exercise skill in sifting through the citations to arrive at the appropriate diagnosis. A recent study found that Google searches revealed the correct diagnosis in 58% of the case records of the *New England Journal of Medicine*,[12] although each search query resulted in many results, which then had to be manually reviewed for appropriateness within the case's context.

Like a traditional diagnostic test, a search can be described by sensitivity, specificity, and the number of articles needed to read.[13] For example, in a study comparing the performance of search strategies to identify clinical practice guidelines in Google Scholar and SUMSearch (another freely accessible search engine), using the term *guideline* yielded the highest sensitivity and using the term *practice guideline* generated the highest specificity and the lowest number of articles needed to read (Table 21.4).[14]

Although there are several other popular hosts of web-based search engines, a more robust decision-support program may help physicians more efficiently consider relevant diagnoses. One program, named *Isabel*, has been developed through the indexing of a database of more than 11,000 diseases according to word patterns in journal articles

TABLE 21.3 Strengths and Weakness of Google Scholar and PubMed

Google Scholar	PubMed
1. Database selection is clumped under subject areas, and it cannot be searched with unique identifiers: Con	1. It allows one to choose a database at the outset and can search with a unique identifier (PubMed identifier): Pro
2. Results cannot be filtered (ie, it does not allow multiple article selection): Con	2. The single citation matcher allows retrieval of articles with pieces of information: Pro
3. A search for related articles or similar pages is not available: Con	3. It allows article selection by checkbox to reduce the number of articles relevant to the search query and to append the filter to search box: Pro
4. It allows one to search by "without" words to exclude unwanted and confusing retrieved data: Pro	4. It provides unique identifier (PubMed identifier) for each retrieved article for easy communicability: Pro
5. It allows one to search a single journal/publication of interest: Pro	5. Searches are limited to journals only; it does not include the gray area of literature: Con
6. Initial search results are those articles that are most cited by journals that themselves are the most cited: Pro	6. It lists search results in chronological order and not by relevance: Con

TABLE 21.4 Retrieval Performance of Search Strategies Using SUMSearch and Google Scholar

Search Strategy	Sensitivity (%)	Specificity (%)	NNR
SUMSearch			
Guideline*	81.51 (74.53–88.49)	74.29 (72.64–75.94)	8.18 (6.90–10.05)
Recommendation*	60.50 (51.72–69.28)	76.28 (74.67–77.89)	9.93 (8.14–12.72)
Practice guideline*	40.34 (31.52–49.16)	89.45 (88.29–90.61)	6.96 (5.52–9.43)
Google Scholar			
Guideline/s	31.93 (23.56–40.30)	78.05 (76.50–79.60)	16.67 (12.76–24.04)
Recommendation/s	8.40 (3.42–13.38)	92.11 (91.09–93.13)	22.42 (13.97–56.82)
Practice guideline/s	11.76 (5.98–17.54)	95.72 (94.96–96.48)	9.29 (6.21–18.38)

NOTE: The 95% confidence intervals are shown in parentheses. This table is reprinted with permission from *BMS Medical Research Methodology*.[14] Copyright 2007, BioMed Central, Ltd.
Abbreviation: NNR, number needed to read.
*Truncation.

associated with each disease, and it is updated as new and relevant articles emerge. One recent study demonstrated that the correct diagnosis was made in 48 of 50 cases (96%) with specific key findings as search terms but in only 37 of the same 50 cases (74%) if the entire case history was simply pasted in, again emphasizing the importance of specific search terms.[15]

POEMS syndrome is a rare entity occasionally seen in middle-aged individuals and marked by a multitude of nonspecific findings, particularly polyneuropathy and plasma cell dyscrasia. In this case, the "diagnostic test" was an Internet search based on the most prominent clinical symptoms. Such a strategy can provide a powerful addition to traditional literature and MEDLINE resources. However, the efficiency of this process is heavily dependent on the quality of the search strategy and, therefore, the cognitive faculties of the treating physician to avoid the predictable shortcoming of low specificity.

"Garbage in, garbage out" still applies, whether the computer in question is the human mind or the desktop PC.

Key Points

1. POEMS syndrome, also known as the *Crow–Fukase syndrome*, is a rare multisystem disorder characterized by polyneuropathy, organomegaly, endocrinopathy, monoclonal gammopathy, and skin changes.
2. Internet searches using search engines such as Google Scholar appear most useful as adjuncts to PubMed and clinical reasoning in identifying case reports when a well-constructed collection of symptoms and signs is used for searches.

REFERENCES

1. Crow RS. Peripheral neuritis in myelomatosis. *Br Med J*. 1956;2(4996):802–804.
2. Bardwick PA, Zvaifler NJ, Gill GN, Newman D, Greenway GD, Resnick DL. Plasma cell dyscrasia with polyneuropathy, organomegaly, endocrinopathy, M protein, and skin changes: the POEMS syndrome. Report on two cases and a review of the literature. *Medicine (Baltimore)*. 1980;59(4):311–322.
3. Osame M. *Nationwide epidemiologic survey of Crow-Fukase syndrome in 2004*. Tokyo, Japan: Japanese Ministry of Health and Welfare Government Report, 2004.
4. Nakanishi T, Sobue I, Toyokura Y, et al. The Crow-Fukase syndrome: A study of 102 cases in Japan. *Neurology*. 1984;34(6):712–720.
5. Soubrier MJ, Dubost JJ, Sauvezie BJ. POEMS syndrome: A study of 25 cases and a review of the literature. French Study Group on POEMS Syndrome. *Am J Med*. 1994;97(6):543–553.
6. Dispenzieri A, Kyle RA, Lacy MQ, et al. POEMS syndrome: Definitions and long-term outcome. *Blood*. 2003;101(7):2496–2506.
7. Dispenzieri A. POEMS syndrome. *Hematology*. 2005;1(1):360–367.
8. Watanabe O, Arimura K, Kitajima I, Osame M, Maruyama I. Greatly raised vascular endothelial growth factor (VEGF) in POEMS syndrome. *Lancet*. 1996;347(9002):702.
9. Henry JA, Altmann IP Assessment of hypoproteinaemic oedema: A simple journal value. *Health Info Libr J*. 2005;22(2):81–82.
10. Koga H, Tokunaga Y, Hisamoto T, et al. Ratio of serum vascular endothelial growth factor to platelet count correlates with disease activity in a patient with POEMS syndrome. *Eur J Intern Med*. 2002;13(1):70–74.
11. Cullen RJ. In search of evidence: Family practitioners' use of the Internet for clinical information. *J Med Libr Assoc*. 2002;90(4):370–379.
12. Tang H, Ng JH. Googling for a diagnosis—use of Google as a diagnostic aid: Internet based study. *BMJ*. 2006;333(7579):1143–5114.
13. Toth B, Gray JA, Brice A. The number needed to read—a new measure of physical sign. *Br Med J*. 1978;1(6117):890–891.
14. Haase A, Markus F, Guido S, Hanna K. Developing search strategies for clinical practice guidelines in SUMSearch and Google Scholar and assessing their retrieval performance. *BMC Med Res Methodol*. 2007;7:28.
15. Graber ML, Mathew A. Performance of a web-based clinical diagnosis support system for internists. *J Gen Intern Med*. 2008;23(Suppl 1):37–40.

CHAPTER 22

IN THE FACE OF IT ALL

AMIT GARG and THOMAS E. BAUDENDISTEL
Department of Medicine, Kaiser Permanente Medical Center, Oakland, California

GURPREET DHALIWAL
Department of Medicine, University of California, San Francisco, California; Medical Service, San Francisco VA Medical Center, San Francisco, California

A 59 year-old man was sent from urgent care clinic to the emergency department for further evaluation because of 1 month of diarrhea and an acute elevation in his serum creatinine.

Whereas acute diarrhea is commonly due to a self-limited and often unspecified infection, diarrhea that extends beyond 2–3 weeks (chronic) warrants consideration of malabsorptive, inflammatory, infectious, and malignant processes. The acute renal failure likely is a consequence of dehydration, but the possibility of simultaneous gastrointestinal and renal involvement from a systemic process (e.g., vasculitis) must be considered.

The patient's diarrhea began 1 month prior, shortly after having a milkshake at a fast-food restaurant. The diarrhea was initially watery, occurred 8–10 times per day, occasionally awakened him at night, and was associated with nausea. There was no mucus, blood, or steatorrhea until 1 day prior to presentation, when he developed epigastric pain and bloody stools. He denied any recent travel outside northern California and had no sick contacts. He had lost 10 pounds over the preceding month. He denied fevers, chills, vomiting, or jaundice, and had not taken antibiotics recently.

In the setting of chronic diarrhea, unintentional weight loss is an alarming feature but does not narrow the diagnostic possibilities significantly. The appearance of blood and pain on a single day after 1 month of symptoms renders their diagnostic value uncertain. For instance, rectal or hemorrhoidal bleeding would be a common occurrence after 1 month of frequent defecation. Sustained bloody stools might be seen in any form of erosive luminal disease, such as infection, inflammatory bowel disease, or neoplasm. Pain is compatible with inflammatory bowel disease, obstructing neoplasms, infections, or ischemia (e.g., vasculitis). There are no fever or chills to support infection, and common gram-negative enteric pathogens (such as *Salmonella, Campylobacter*, and *Yersinia*) usually do not produce symptoms for such an extended period. He has not taken antibiotics, which would predispose him to infection with *Clostridium difficile*, and he has no obvious exposure to parasites such as *Entamoeba*.

The patient had diabetes mellitus with microalbuminuria, chronic obstructive pulmonary disease, hypertension, hyperlipidemia, chronic low-back pain, and

Clinical Care Conundrums: Challenging Diagnoses in Hospital Medicine, First Edition.
Edited by James C. Pile, Thomas E. Baudendistel, and Brian J. Harte.

gastritis, and had undergone a Billroth II procedure for a perforated gastric ulcer in the past. His medications included omeprazole, insulin glargine, simvastatin, lisinopril, amlodipine, and albuterol- and beclomethasone-metered dose inhalers. He had been married for 31 years, lived at home with his wife, was a former rigger in a shipyard, and was on disability for chronic low-back pain. He denied alcohol or intravenous drug use but had quit tobacco 5 years prior after more than 40 pack-years of smoking. He had three healthy adult children and there was no family history of cancer, liver disease, or inflammatory bowel disease. There was no history of sexually transmitted diseases or unprotected sexual intercourse.

Bacterial overgrowth in the blind loop following a Billroth II operation can lead to malabsorption, but the diarrhea would not begin so abruptly this long after surgery. Medications are common causes of diarrhea. Proton pump inhibitors, by reducing gastric acidity, confer an increased risk of bacterial enteritis; they also are a risk factor for *C. difficile*. Lisinopril may cause bowel angioedema months or years after initiation. Occult laxative use is a well-recognized cause of chronic diarrhea and should also be considered. The most relevant element of his social history is the prolonged smoking and the attendant risk of cancer, although diarrhea is a rare paraneoplastic phenomenon.

On exam, temperature was 36.6°C; blood pressure, 125/78 mm Hg; pulse, 88; respiratory rate, 16 per minute; and oxygen saturation, 97% while breathing room air. There was temporal wasting and mild scleral icterus, but no jaundice. Lungs were clear to auscultation and heart was regular in rate and rhythm without murmurs or gallops. There was no jugular venous distention. A large abdominal midline scar was present, bowel sounds were normoactive, and the abdomen was soft, nontender, and nondistended. The liver edge was 6 cm below the costal margin; there was no splenomegaly. The patient was alert and oriented, with a normal neurologic exam.

The liver generally enlarges because of acute inflammation, congestion, or infiltration. Infiltration can be due to tumors, infections, hemochromatosis, amyloidosis, or sarcoidosis. A normal cardiac exam argues against hepatic congestion from right-sided heart failure or pericardial disease.

The key elements of the case are diarrhea and hepatomegaly. Inflammatory bowel disease can be accompanied by sclerosing cholangitis, but this should not enlarge the liver. Mycobacterial infections and syphilis can infiltrate the liver and intestinal mucosa, causing diarrhea, but he lacks typical risk factors.

Malignancy is an increasing concern. Colon cancer commonly metastasizes to the liver and can occasionally be intensely secretory. Pancreatic cancer could account for these symptoms, especially if pancreatic exocrine insufficiency caused malabsorption. Various rare neuroendocrine tumors that arise in the pancreas can cause secretory diarrheas and liver metastases, such as carcinoid, VIPoma, and the Zollinger–Ellison syndrome.

Laboratory results revealed a serum sodium of 143 mmol/L, potassium of 4.7 mmol/L, chloride of 110 mmol/L, bicarbonate of 25 mmol/L, urea nitrogen of 24 mg/dL, and creatinine of 2.5 mg/dL (baseline had been 1.2 mg/dL 2 months previously). Serum glucose was 108 mg/dL and calcium was 8.8 mg/dL. The total white blood cell count was 9300/mm^3 with a normal differential, hemoglobin was 14.4 g/dL, mean corpuscular volume was 87 fL, and the platelet count was normal. Total bilirubin was 3.7 mg/dL, and direct bilirubin was 3.1 mg/dL. Aspartate aminotransferase (AST) was 122 U/L (normal range, 8–31), alanine aminotransferase (ALT) 79 U/L (normal range, 7–31), alkaline phosphatase 1591 U/L (normal range, 39–117), and

gamma-glutamyltransferase (GGT) 980 U/L (normal range, <57). Serum albumin was 2.5 mg/dL, prothrombin time was 16.4 seconds, and international normalized ratio (INR) was 1.6.

Urinalysis was normal except for trace hemoglobin, small bilirubin, and 70 mg/dL of protein; specific gravity was 1.007. Urine microscopy demonstrated no cells or casts. The ratio of protein to creatinine on a spot urine sample was less than 1. Chest X-ray was normal. The electrocardiogram demonstrated sinus rhythm with an old right bundle branch block and normal QRS voltages.

The disproportionate elevation in alkaline phosphatase points to an infiltrative hepatopathy from a cancer originating in the gastrointestinal tract or infection. Other infiltrative processes such as sarcoidosis or amyloidosis usually have evidence of disease elsewhere before hepatic disease becomes apparent.

Mild proteinuria may be explained by diabetes. The specific gravity of 1.007 is atypical for dehydration and could suggest ischemic tubular injury. Although intrinsic renal diseases must continue to be entertained, hypovolemia (compounded by angiotensin-converting enzyme [ACE] inhibitor use) is the leading explanation in light of the nondiagnostic renal studies. The preserved hemoglobin may simply indicate dehydration, but otherwise is somewhat reassuring in the context of bloody diarrhea.

The patient was admitted to the hospital. Three stool samples returned negative for *C. difficile* toxin. No white cells were detected in the stool, and no ova or parasites were detected. Stool culture was negative for routine bacterial pathogens and for *Escherichia coli* O157. Tests for human immunodeficiency virus and antinuclear antibodies (ANAs) and serologies for hepatitis A, B, and C were negative. Abdominal ultrasound demonstrated no intra- or extrahepatic bile duct dilatation; no hepatic masses were seen. Kidneys were normal in size and appearance without hydronephrosis. Computed tomography (CT) of the abdomen without intravenous contrast revealed normal-appearing liver (with a 12-cm span), spleen, biliary ducts, and pancreas, and there was no intra-abdominal adenopathy.

The stool studies point away from infectious colitis. Infiltrative processes of the liver, including metastases, lymphoma, tuberculosis, syphilis, amyloidosis, and sarcoidosis, can be microscopic and therefore evade detection by ultrasound and CT scan. In conditions such as these, endoscopic retrograde cholangiopancreatography (ERCP)/magnetic resonance cholangiopancreatography (MRCP) or liver biopsy may be required. CT is limited without contrast but does not suggest extrahepatic disease in the abdomen.

MRCP was performed, but was a technically suboptimal study due to the presence of ascites. The serum creatinine improved to 1.4 mg/dL over the next 4 days, and the patient's diarrhea decreased to two bowel movements daily with the use of loperamide. The patient was discharged home with outpatient gastroenterology follow-up planned to discuss further evaluation of the abnormal liver enzymes.

Prior to being seen in the gastroenterology clinic, the patient's nonbloody diarrhea worsened. He felt weaker and continued to lose weight. He also noted new onset of bilateral lower face numbness and burning, which was followed by swelling of his lower lip 12 hours later. He returned to the hospital.

On examination, he was afebrile. His lower lip was markedly swollen and was drooping from his face. He could not move the lip to close his mouth. The upper lip and tongue were normal in size and moved without restriction. Facial sensation was intact, but there was weakness when he attempted to wrinkle both of his brows and close his eyelids. The rest of his physical examination was unchanged.

The serum creatinine had risen to 3.6 mg/dL, and the complete blood count remained normal. Serum total bilirubin was 4.6 mg/dL; AST, 87 U/L; ALT, 76 U/L; and alkaline phosphatase, 1910 U/L. The 24-hour urine protein measurement was 86 mg.

Lip swelling suggests angioedema. ACE inhibitors are frequent offenders, and it would be important to know whether his lisinopril was restarted at discharge. ACE-inhibitor angioedema can also affect the intestine, causing abdominal pain and diarrhea, but does not cause a systemic wasting illness or infiltrative hepatopathy. The difficulty moving the lip may reflect the physical effects of swelling, but generalized facial weakness supports a cranial neuropathy. Basilar meningitis may produce multiple cranial neuropathies, the etiologies of which are quite similar to the previously mentioned causes of infiltrative liver disease: sarcoidosis, syphilis, tuberculosis, or lymphoma.

The patient had not resumed lisinopril since his prior hospitalization. The lower lip swelling and paralysis persisted, and new sensory paresthesias developed over the right side of his chin. A consulting neurologist found normal language and speech and moderate dysarthria. Cranial nerve exam was normal except for the bilateral lower motor neuron facial nerve palsy that was noted with bilateral facial droop, reduced strength of eyelid closure, and diminished forehead movement bilaterally; facial sensation was normal. Extremity motor exam revealed proximal iliopsoas muscle weakness bilaterally rated as 4/5 and was otherwise normal. Sensation to pinprick was diminished in a stocking/glove distribution. Deep-tendon reflexes were normal and plantar response was downgoing bilaterally. Coordination was intact, Romberg was negative, and gait was slowed due to weakness.

Over the next several days, the patient continued to have diarrhea and facial symptoms. The serum total bilirubin increased to 14 mg/dL, alkaline phosphatase rose above 2000 U/L, and serum creatinine increased to 5.5 mg/dL. Noncontrast CT scan of the head was normal.

Along with a mild peripheral sensory neuropathy, the exam indicates bilateral palsies of the facial nerve. Lyme disease is a frequent etiology, but this patient is not from an endemic area. I am most suspicious of bilateral infiltration of cranial nerve VII. I am thinking analogically to the numb chin syndrome (NCS), wherein lymphoma or breast cancer infiltration along the mental branch of V3 causes sensory loss, and perhaps these disorders can produce infiltrative facial neuropathy. At this point, I am most concerned about lymphomatous meningitis with cranial nerve involvement. Cerebrospinal fluid (CSF) analysis (including cytology) would be informative.

Lumbar puncture demonstrated clear CSF with one white blood cell per mm^3 and no red blood cells. Glucose was normal, and protein was 95.5 (normal range, 15–45 mg/dL). Gram stain and culture for bacteria were negative, as were polymerase chain reaction (PCR) testing for herpes simplex virus, mycobacterial and fungal stains and cultures, and cytology. Transthoracic echocardiogram demonstrated severe concentric left ventricular (LV) hypertrophy, normal LV systolic function, and impaired LV relaxation. CT scan of the chest identified no adenopathy or other abnormalities.

The CSF analysis does not support basilar meningitis, although the cytoalbuminologic dissociation makes me wonder whether there is some intrathecal antibody production or an autoimmune process we have yet to uncover. The absence of lymphadenopathy anywhere in the body and the negative CSF cytology now point away from lymphoma. As the case for lymphoma or an infection diminishes, systemic amyloidosis rises to the top of possibilities in this afebrile man who is losing weight and

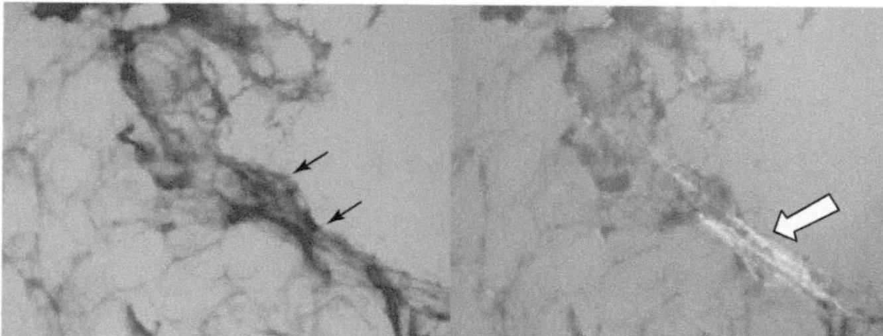

FIGURE 22.1 Fat pad biopsy: congophilic (black arrows) and apple-green birefringent material (white arrow) associated with blood vessels indicative of amyloid.

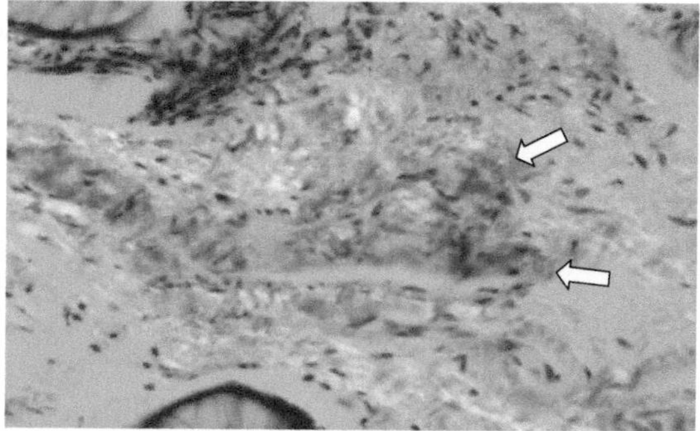

FIGURE 22.2 Rectal biopsy: congophilic material within blood vessels consistent with amyloid. Magnification: 169 × 105 mm (96 × 96 DPI).

has an infiltrative liver and nerve abnormalities, renal failure, cardiac enlargement, and suspected gastrointestinal luminal abnormality. Although the echocardiographic findings are most likely explained by hypertension, they are compatible with amyloid infiltration. A tissue specimen is needed, and either colonoscopy or liver biopsy should be suitable.

A pathologist performed a fat pad biopsy that demonstrated scant congophilic and birefringent material associated with blood vessels, suggestive of amyloid (Fig. 22.1). Colonoscopy demonstrated normal mucosa, and a rectal biopsy revealed congophilic material within the blood vessels consistent with amyloid (Fig. 22.2). No monoclonal band was present on serum protein electrophoresis. Urine protein electrophoresis identified a homogenous band in the gamma region, and urine kappa and lambda free light chains were increased: kappa was 10.7 mg/dL (normal range, <2) and lambda was 4.25 mg/dL (normal range, <2).

After an extensive discussion among the patient, his wife, and a palliative care physician, the patient declined chemotherapy and elected to go home. Two days after discharge (7 weeks after his initial admission for diarrhea) he died in his sleep at home. Permission for a postmortem examination was not granted.

DISCUSSION

Amyloidosis refers to abnormal extracellular deposition of fibril. There are many types of amyloidosis including primary amyloidosis (AL amyloidosis), secondary amyloidosis (AA amyloidosis), and hereditary causes. Systemic AL amyloidosis is a rare plasma cell

TABLE 22.1 Common Findings in Primary (AL) Amyloidosis*

Organ Involvement	Incidence of Organ Involvement (%)	Symptoms	Signs	Laboratory/Test Finding
General	—	Malaise, weight loss	—	—
Renal	33	Fatigue	Peripheral edema	Proteinuria with or without renal insufficiency, pleural effusion, hypercholesterolemia
Cardiac	20	Palpitations, dyspnea	Elevated jugular venous pressure, S3, peripheral edema, hepatomegaly	Low-voltage or atrial fibrillation on electrocardiogram; echocardiogram shows thickened ventricles and dilated atria
Neurological	20	Paresthesias, numbness, weakness, autonomic insufficiency	Carpal tunnel syndrome, postural hypotension	—
Gastrointestinal and hepatic	16	Diarrhea, nausea, weight loss	Macroglossia, hepatomegaly	Elevated alkaline phosphatase
Hematology	Rare	Bleeding	Periorbital purpura (raccoon eyes)	Prolonged prothrombin time, factor X deficiency

*See reference 2.

disorder characterized by misfolding of insoluble extracellular fibrillar proteins derived from immunoglobulin light chains. These insoluble proteins typically deposit in the kidney, heart, and nervous system.[1] Although the mechanism of organ dysfunction is debated, deposition of these proteins may disrupt the tissue architecture by interacting with local receptors and causing apoptosis.[1]

Table 22.1 indicates the most common findings in patients with AL amyloidosis.[2] Although our patient ultimately developed many common findings of AL amyloidosis, several features were atypical, including the marked hyperbilirubinemia, profound diarrhea, and bilateral facial diplegia.

Up to 70% of patients with amyloidosis will have detectable liver deposits, typically involving portal vessels, portal stroma, central vein, and sinusoidal parenchyma.[3] Clinically overt hepatic dysfunction from amyloid is less frequent,[4] and the most characteristic findings are hepatomegaly with a markedly elevated serum alkaline phosphatase concentration; jaundice is rare. Palpable hepatic enlargement without abnormal liver enzymes should be interpreted with caution. The finding of a palpable liver edge correlates poorly with frank hepatomegaly, with a positive likelihood ratio of just 1.7.[5] In the patient under discussion, suspected hepatomegaly was not confirmed on a subsequent CT scan. Nonetheless, the elevated alkaline phosphatase represented an important clue to potential infiltrative liver disease. In a series of amyloidosis patients from the Mayo Clinic, 81% had hepatomegaly on physical exam and the mean alkaline phosphatase level was 1029 U/L (normal, <250 U/L), while the mean serum bilirubin and AST levels were only modestly elevated, at 3.2 mg/dL and 72 U/L, respectively. The prothrombin time was prolonged in 35% of patients.

Upper gastrointestinal tract involvement by AL amyloid may be found in up to one-third of cases at autopsy, but clinically significant gastrointestinal features are seen in fewer than 5% of patients.[6] Predominant intestinal manifestations are unintentional weight loss (average 7 kg) and diarrhea, nonspecific features that result in delayed diagnosis for a median of 7 months after symptom onset.[7] Diarrhea in AL amyloid may stem from several mechanisms: small intestine mucosal infiltration, steatorrhea from pancreatic insufficiency, autonomic neuropathy leading to pseudo-obstruction and bacterial overgrowth, bile acid malabsorption, or rapid transit time. Diarrhea in AL amyloid is often resistant to treatment and may be the primary cause of death.[7]

Systemic amyloidosis commonly produces peripheral neuropathies. Involvement of small unmyelinated fibers causes paresthesias and progressive sensory loss in a pattern that is usually distal, symmetric, and progressive.[6,8] Our patient presented with bilateral sensory paresthesias of the chin, suggesting the NCS that is characterized by facial numbness along the distribution of the mental branch of the trigeminal nerve. While dental disorders and infiltration from malignant tumors (mostly lung and breast cancer) account for most cases, amyloidosis and other infiltrative disorders are also known to cause NCS.[9,10] Our patient's sensory paresthesias may have represented amyloid infiltration of peripheral nerves.

With the exception of carpal tunnel syndrome, motor or cranial neuropathy is uncommon in amyloid, and when present usually heralds advanced disease.[11] Descriptions of bilateral facial weakness, also known as *facial diplegia*, from amyloidosis are limited to case reports.[12–14] Other causes of this rare finding include sarcoidosis, Guillain–Barre syndrome, and Lyme disease.[15]

The diagnosis of primary amyloidosis requires histologic evidence of amyloid from a tissue biopsy specimen (demonstrating positive Congo red staining and pathognomonic green birefringence under cross-polarized light microscopy), and the presence of a clonal plasma cell disorder. While biopsy of an affected organ is diagnostic, more easily obtained samples such as fat pad biopsy and rectal biopsy yield positive results in up to 80% of cases.[2] Serum and urine protein electrophoresis with immunofixation identifies an underlying plasma cell disorder in 90% of cases of primary amyloidosis. When these tests are inconclusive, serum or urine free light chain assays or bone marrow aspirate and biopsy are useful aids to detect underlying plasma cell dyscrasia.[2] AL amyloidosis is a progressive disease with median survival of about 1–2 years.[16] Poorer prognosis is associated with substantial echocardiographic findings, autonomic neuropathy, and liver involvement.[2] Hyperbilirubinemia is associated with a poor prognosis, with a median survival of 8.5 months.[4] Proteinuria or peripheral neuropathy portends a less ominous course.[6]

Treatment goals include reducing production and deposition of fibril proteins and contending with organ dysfunction (eg, congestive heart failure management). Selected patients with AL amyloidosis may be candidates for high-dose melphalan and autologous stem cell transplantation.

It would not be reasonable for clinicians to suspect amyloidosis in cases of diarrhea until two conditions are met: (i) the absence of evidence for the typical etiologies of diarrhea and (ii) the evolving picture of an infiltrative disorder. The latter was heralded by the elevated alkaline phosphatase and was supported by the subsequent multiorgan involvement. Conceptualizing the disease as "infiltrative" still required a diligent exclusion of infection and invasive tumor cells, which invade disparate organs far more commonly than amyloidosis. Their absence and the organ pattern that is typical of AL amyloidosis (heart, kidney, and peripheral nerve involvement) allowed the discussant to reason by analogy that amyloidosis was also responsible for the most symptomatic phenomena, namely, diarrhea and facial diplegia (and NCS).

Key Points

1. Hospitalists should consider systemic amyloidosis in cases of unexplained diarrhea when other clinical features of AL amyloidosis are present, including nephrotic syndrome with or without renal insufficiency, cardiomyopathy, peripheral neuropathy, and hepatomegaly.
2. Hepatic amyloidosis should be suspected when weight loss, hepatomegaly, and elevated alkaline phosphatase are present. Although jaundice is rare in amyloidosis, liver involvement and hyperbilirubinemia portend a poorer prognosis.
3. NCS and bilateral facial diplegia are rare manifestations of AL amyloid deposition in peripheral nerves.

REFERENCES

1. Merlini G, Bellotti V. Molecular mechanisms of amyloidosis. *N Engl J Med*. 2003;349(6):583–596.
2. Guidelines Working Group of UK Myeloma Forum; British Committee for Standards in Haematology, British Society for Haematology. Guidelines on the diagnosis and management of AL amyloidosis. *Br J Haematol*. 2004;125:681–700.
3. Buck FS, Koss MN. Hepatic amyloidosis: Morphologic differences between systemic AL and AA types. *Hum Pathol*. 1991;22(9):904–907.
4. Park MA, Mueller PS, Kyle RA, et al. Primary (AL) hepatic amyloidosis clinical features and natural history in 98 patients. *Medicine*. 2003;82(5):291–298.
5. McGee S. *Evidence-based physical diagnosis*. Philadelphia, PA: WB Saunders; 2001:595–599.
6. Gertz MA, Comenzo R, Falk RH, et al. Definition of organ involvement and treatment response in immunoglobulin light chain amyloidosis (AL): A consensus opinion from the 10th International Symposium on Amyloid and Amyloidosis. *Am J Hematol*. 2005;79:319–328.
7. Madsen LG. Primary (AL) amyloidosis with gastrointestinal involvement. *Scand J Gastroenterol*. 2009;44(6):708–711.
8. Kyle RA, Gertz MA. Primary systemic amyloidosis: Clinical and laboratory features in 474 cases. *Semin Hematol*. 1995;32:45–59.
9. Colella G, Giudice A, Siniscalchi G, Falcone U, Guastafierro S. Chin numbness: A symptom that should not be underestimated: A review of 12 cases. *Am J Med Sci*. 2009;337:407–410.
10. Marinella MA. Numb chin syndrome: A subtle clue to possible serious illness. *Hosp Physician*. 2000;36:54–56.
11. Freeman R. Autonomic peripheral neuropathy. *Neurol Clin*. 2007;25:277–301.
12. Massey EW, Massey JM. Facial diplegia due to amyloidosis. *South Med J*. 1986;79(11):1458–1459.
13. Darras BT, Adelman LS, Mora JS, Bodziner RA, Munsat TL. Familial amyloidosis with cranial neuropathy and corneal lattice dystrophy. *Neurology*. 1986;36:432–435.
14. Traynor AE, Gertz MA, Kyle RA. Crainal neuropathy associated with primary amyloidosis. *Ann Neurol*. 1991;29:451–454.
15. Keane JR. Bilateral seventh nerve palsy: Analysis of 43 cases and review of the literature. *Neurology*. 1994;44:1198–202.
16. Ebert EC, Nagar M. Gastrointestinal manifestations of amyloid. *Am J Gastroenterol*. 2008;103:776–787.

INDEX

Clinical Care Conundrums: Challenging Diagnoses in Hospital Medicine, First Edition.
Edited by James C. Pile, Thomas E. Baudendistel, and Brian J. Harte.